COMPACTS

POWDER, AN

WITH VALUES

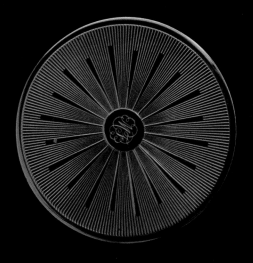

FRANCES JOHNSON

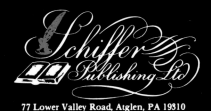

Schiffer Publishing Ltd

77 Lower Valley Road, Atglen, PA 19310

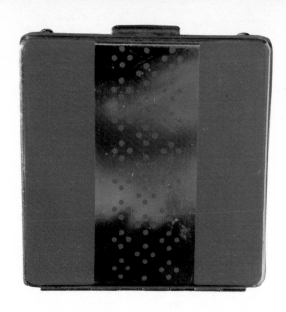

Printed in Hong Kong
ISBN: 0-7643-0055-5

Library of Congress
Cataloging-in-Publication Data

Johnson, Frances.
  Compacts, powder, and paint/Frances
Johnson.
    p. cm.
  ISBN 0-7643-0055-5
  1. Compacts (Cosmetics)--Collectors and
collecting--Catalogs. 2. Compacts (Cosmetics)-
-History. I. Title.
NK4890.C65J64   1996
745.593--dc20   96-7590
                                               CIP

Published by Schiffer Publishing, Ltd.
77 Lower Valley Road
Atglen, PA 19310
Please write for a free catalog.
This book may be purchased from the publisher.
Please include $2.95 postage.
Try your bookstore first.

We are interested in hearing from authors
with book ideas on related subjects.

Contents

Introduction

There is still a plentiful supply of compacts available today—some elegant, others more plain and cheap than elegant, and most available for a price collectors can afford. This is due, no doubt, to the fact that during the thirties through the sixties, people lived in a completely different social environment than we live in today. During these years, the majority of mothers stayed home, and they also made strict rules by which children had to abide, especially girls. Most girls were not allowed to date until they were sixteen or older, unless of course they slipped around and the mother didn't find out. Another strict rule concerned gifts from boyfriends. Only four items—flowers, candy, perfume, or a compact—were acceptable. At least 98 percent of the mothers enforced this ruling, and everyone abided by it. Gifts other than these four were considered too personal, while anything remotely relating to clothing caused mothers to swoon, probably a carry-over from the staid Victorian era.

The compact was the most popular of these gifts. It would also last longer. Flowers would die, candy be eaten, and perfume used, but the compact continued to be used for years. Compacts were also favorite gifts for girls to give each other, for husbands to give wives, and parents to give to their daughters. One of the reasons for their lasting popularity was because they were useful. Girls had always used cosmetics, sometimes sparingly and other times quite generously, but they never quit using them entirely. The compact meant they could take their makeup with them to repair any "damage."

The automobile can be credited with adding to the popularity of the compact. Now boys could take girls out for dinner, or maybe dinner and dancing. After a meal she naturally needed to check her makeup. Here we find the origin of another social code, probably left over from some misguided interpretation of Victorian etiquette. The accepted norm was that a girl must never, under any circumstances, repair her makeup at the table in a restaurant, or in any public place. But with the increasing popularity of the compact and perhaps the excessive use of it as a gift, the rules were relaxed a bit. After the young lady had thanked her boyfriend profusely for an elegant compact, it was feared he might not know for sure whether or not she really liked it; therefore she was allowed to remove it from her purse when they were dining out, open it briefly to check her makeup. This assured him she did like it and was using it. She could then go to the powder room and repair her makeup. Oh! the games people used to play. Today's honesty is so refreshing.

A note on prices in this book—the following prices have been gathered from various sources and locations. Since compacts are such a new collectible, prices have not yet begun to stabilize, so it is sort of a guessing game as to the perfect price for each one in each location. If you find one you really like at a price you can afford, we suggest you buy it. Chances are the price will triple within the next five years.

Chapter One:
The Story of Powder and Paint

Nobody seems to know where the term "Painted Hussy" originated, but chances are it began in the twenties when the Flappers of that period tried to imitate movie stars who used lots of makeup. (Like everything else in the world the word *hussy* can also be controversial—my dictionary gives two very different meanings: First, a saucy or flippant girl, second, a strumpet; trollop. The term was used at different times in history to describe various people, but chances are when it was used in the twenties it wasn't used to describe a saucy, flippant girl). Of course the Flappers probably did use too much makeup, but for the first time in this century young women not only had someone to lead them, their leaders were also movie stars. On the silver screen young women could see how to use the makeup and how pretty the stars who used it were. Not only did the movie stars use lots of powder and paint, but for the next thirty years or so they could be found in many of the women's magazines, in full page ads, praising first one and then another cosmetic company's products. Admittedly, throughout the years some women have gone overboard and used too much makeup, but I doubt they could have looked much worse than some of the women in the past, especially the Egyptians of six to eight centuries ago. The custom then was to powder the face stark white, while painting their eyebrows and lashes black and their cheeks red. During this period they used a blue-black lipstick. I imagine all of this color against such a chalky white face must have been frightening indeed.

This alone might explain why there has been so much controversy over the use of woman's makeup since its very beginning—about eight thousand years ago. Throughout history men have used cosmetics, sometimes as much or more than women, yet they have tried to control women's use of makeup with both name calling at times and with legislation at others. Neither method seemed to work, but they did try. An example of this can be found as early as the second century when a Greek theologian named Clement worked to implement a law which would "prevent women from tricking men into marriage with the use of cosmetics." Two centuries later, another Greek wrote about how disappointed he was when he found his new wife had deceived him by "painting" herself. He wrote that he tried to explain to her that the act was as dishonest as if he had tried to deceive her about his property. This vendetta between men and women over the use of cosmetics continued until about 1770 when a law was introduced and defeated in the British Parliament stating that women, regardless of age, rank, or profession or whether or not they were virgins, maids, or widows, would be tried for witchcraft and have their marriage terminated if the woman had "seduced or betrayed [a man] into marriage by the use of scents, paints, cosmetic washes, artificial teeth, or false hair." Wigs were big and commonly used in those days.

But it wasn't all fussing and fighting. Around 4000 B.C. the Egyptians, both men and women, were among the best coifed and well painted in the known world. Of course the world wasn't nearly as large as it is now, but there were still quite a few people. From research it seems all of Egypt made and used cosmetics, heavily. Not only did they use their powders and paints lavishly, they kept large supplies to be buried with them so they would have plenty in their next life. Surprisingly, some of the same colors they used then are still popular. For instance, they preferred green eye shadow they made or had made by grinding green copper ore into a powder. Some cream or oil had to be added so it could be applied heavily. They didn't seem to use any of their cosmetics sparingly perhaps in the belief that if a little would help, a lot would make them beautiful. The Egyptians were also the first to use glittery eye shadow. To obtain this fancy cosmetic they ground the iridescent shells of some beetles and added this mixture to the green eye shadow.

Some people have long thought the eyes were the most expressive part of the face—that they revealed the innermost thoughts of the person. Maybe this theory originated with the Egyptians as they seemed to believe the eyes deserved lots of makeup. Anyone who has seen movies of the early Egyptians will remember the heavy eye makeup. Perhaps more interesting than the heavy green eye shadow was the heavier mascara. It is doubtful they actually called it mascara, but it was a black paste made of burnt almonds, black oxide of copper, and brown clay ocher. This mixture was applied heavily to the eyebrows and lashes. The excess was stored in kohl pots for future use. Keep in mind at this time one had to make his or her own makeup, although beauty shops and perfume factories were known centuries before the birth of Christ. It is possible the Egyptians could have bought some of their makeup, although no mention of it being for sale has been found. It is generally believed the servants made most of the cosmetics used in the very early days.

According to old records it appears the Romans did use some makeup, but from all indications they preferred a more natural appearance. In those very early days they seem to be more interested in scholastic and athletic pursuits than in social affairs. Roman women may have used some makeup, but certainly nothing like that used by the Egyptians. And there didn't seem to be nearly as much controversy because men was considered to be king, at least in their own households, while woman were simply their chattel.

One of the reasons behind the friction between male and female over the use of powder and paint could have come from the actions of Jezebel, the wife of Ahab. She introduced eye makeup to the Jewish women when she arrived from Phoenicia around 850 B. C. Phoenicia was a center of fashion at that time so she naturally brought the newest styles and fashions with her. Jezebel's total disregard for everyone's rights didn't make her very popular, nor did her defiance of the Hebrew prophets. Perhaps because she was so heavily made up all the time, she gave cosmetics a bad name. For years the name Jezebel took precedent over the descriptive "Painted Hussy."

Despite all the friction and controversy, powder and paint has survived, and today it is probably one of the most lucrative businesses in the world. We still go through periods of heavy makeup to periods of almost none at all. The twenties were one of the more heavily applied cosmetic periods, then in the thirties many women began sporting a more natural look. The latter could have been cause by the Depression, when women simply didn't have money for cosmetics. This trend continued until the early forties when women went to work for the war effort which gave them money to spend, and they wanted to look nice for their boyfriends. Again cosmetics were used sometimes heavily, other times sparingly. In the fifties and sixties the women seem to layer on the cosmetics. It was applied heavily in many cases. This off again, on again application continues today. In some areas and by some women cosmetics are more heavily used than in others, but never has there been a time when their use was discontinued completely.

Chapter Two:
The Story of the Compact

The compact is believed to have evolved from the patch box designed for another beauty aid. During the 1600s the dreaded and disfiguring disease of smallpox had swept through Europe and the ones who lived through it were left with faces and bodies marred by scars. To cover these scars they began using the so-called "beauty patches," a custom which lasted for a century or more—much longer than the people who were scarred. These patches became so popular that both men and women apparently began to believe they were really patches to enhance their beauty, so the public continued to wear them. At first the patches were cut from black silk or velvet in the shape of hearts, stars, and crescent moons. Then they were placed strategically on the face, lips, throat, and breast, wherever they were needed to cover the scars. Like many other fashions, they continued to be popular for years. It isn't surprising that both men and women wore them, because both sexes had been scarred by smallpox.

Extra patches were always made to replace any that might be lost while one was out in public or at a dance or party, and this created the need for a container that eventually became known as a "patch box." Some of these boxes were absolutely exquisite. They could be made of gold, silver, bone, ivory, tortoiseshell, or any other material one desired. They usually had a small mirror in the top and could have been studded with precious or semi-precious stones. Again we have to bear in mind that although smallpox had disfigured thousands of people, only the nobility and the very rich were invited to balls and parties where it was imperative they cover their scars. The masses could and did cover their scars, but probably not as elegantly as the rich, and it is doubtful they could afford the bejeweled patch boxes. Chances are they had plainer ones. When patches were no longer worn it is believed the patch box served as a model for the compact. But there was a lot of water over the dam before that happened.

One reason for the popularity of beauty patches after they were no longer used to cover the scars was the fact they gave the women who were supposed to be quite shy and who lived in what was described as a well chaperoned society a chance to flirt—outrageously. A correctly positioned patch could send a message to the opposite sex. For instance, it was said that if the woman wore a patch near her mouth, she was flirting. A patch on the right cheek meant she was married, while one on the left cheek indicated she was engaged. And apparently neither commitment had a lot of effect on her flirting—or maybe her affairs. A patch at the corner of the eye denoted smoldering passion, an emotion ladies were not supposed to admit, especially in public. Later, after the patches faded into history, the women used handkerchiefs and fans to send approximately the same messages.

In the very early days powder had been made of carbonate of lead that left the face with what looked like a white mask, but by the twenties the powder was being developed in laboratories. Along with white (not the stark white of the past, but a very pale shade of white) there were several shades of face powder. Each was supposed to fit the needs of the women regardless of whether their complexion was light or dark. The early rouge had come in one shade—red. This is understandable, as we know that the ingredients were mulberry and seaweed, ground to a paste and colored with cinnabar. This also changed by the twenties. And no longer were the women forced to use the dark, one shade lipstick. Now they had several colors from which to choose.

Not only did all types of cosmetics become available during the twenties, but compacts were also being developed. In the beginning most were small and simple, holding only loose or pressed powder and a puff. They all had mirrors, regardless of the style or size. Later rouge and lipstick would be added, then a comb, and finally the carryalls, which became very popular. Some compacts were so elaborate they contained powder, rouge, lipstick, a comb, money compartment, and a cigarette case. A few even had a cigarette lighter. Most had the mirror in the top or one was built in between some of the other features. A few had mirrors that could be pulled out of a thick top. The servicemen in World War II continued the old rule that it was safe to give a girl a compact, and sent millions home from the PXs around the world. In some of these the mirror could be pulled out, and there was a place for *his* picture. It was a great idea, he thought, as it kept his face before her while he was away.

Compared to other antiques and collectibles, the price of compacts is quite reasonable today. Perhaps that stems from the fact most of them were so inexpensive in the twenties and thirties, and even into the forties. At that time plain, run-of-the-mill types could be bought in the ten cent stores of that era for 10 to 25 cents each. The better ones in these stores could run as high as 39 to 49 cents each. Some of those living in rural areas who seldom went to town found it more convenient to order their compacts from mail order houses like Sears, Roebuck and Montgomery Ward. Nearly all the mail order houses at that time offered compacts. An example was Gimbel Brothers, Philadelphia who in 1925 offered compacts made by three different companies. A single Melba compact (powder only) was offered for $1 while a double one with both powder and rouge was priced $1.50. They also offered two pretty but differently shaped double compacts they called Vanities. Then as now each company tried to glamorize their products by giving them fancy names. This has contributed to the confusion over the correct names by which compacts should be known. Like the companies did, we may call them by whatever name sounds best to us. Gimbel's vanities trademarked Karess were priced $1.75. In the same catalog they offered a thin Tre-Jur for 50 cents, a slightly larger one for $1, and a "purse-size twin" (double compact) for $1.25.

Perhaps other companies offered different types of compacts, but we are limited to the available catalogs for types and dates. By 1927 Sears, Roebuck and Company was offering several pages of compacts. No manufacturers were mentioned, but prices varied from 85 cents to $11.75 so they must have been the better known brands.

The popularity of the compact was on the move. With the country in a deep recession in 1932, one wholesale jeweler, Wallenstein Mayer Company, Cincinnati, was offering a compact for $24, and this was the wholesale price. It was described as "Green gold finish, sterling silver top, very thin model, genuine Cloisonné enamel front and back, genuine hand-painted reproduction of the famous Lancret's 'Music Lesson'. Fitted with large mirror, patented Evans' Tap-sift loose powder container, full size rouge, French enamel stone set lipstick handle. In attractive Velveteen covered and lined gift box." Most merchants did not work on the margin of profit used today because their expenses were much less, but they would have had to have at least a $10 mark-up which would have meant the compact was priced at around $35, a tidy sum in a depression. Movie stars could and did buy some very expensive items during this time, and compacts like this one would probably have appealed to them. Not all the compacts in Wallenstein Mayer's catalogue that year were so expensive, several were priced as low as $1.15.

Apparently the depression had not affected the compact business, as Wallenstein Mayer had nine pages of compacts in their catalog in 1932, most of them made by Evans. But compacts were offered from other manufacturers like J. M. Fisher Company, Attleboro, Massachusetts. That year Wallenstein Mayer showed six beautifully enameled examples from that manufacturer. All had chain handles which made them look like very small purses. Wholesale prices on these averaged around $5 each which meant they would sell for around $7 to $9, still a tidy sum for the average woman during that time.

The catalog included two pages of compacts, in color, from McRae & Keller Company. Wholesale prices on these ranged from $2.50 to $5 each. One page was devoted to the "New Whoopee compact that was fitted with an adjustable swinging handle." There was a suggestion offered for its use. The manufacturers said that by fitting the handle over the first three fingers of the left hand, the mirror could be held at just the right angle, or if this method was not satisfactory, the handle could be used as a stand.

Two pages of the catalog were devoted to Volupté compacts, but the ones shown were rather plain for this company. We do find some plain Volupté examples today, but many of us tend to think of them as being rather elaborate. Wholesale prices on these ranged from $1.80 for a simple compact to $4 for one with a lipstick fastened to the chain handle.

Surprisingly, few compacts were found in the early Ovington catalogs. Ovington was one of the more exclusive gift shops on New York's Fifth Avenue, but apparently in 1925 their compact trade was limited mostly to the walk-in trade, as only one compact was offered in their catalog that year. It was a sterling silver vanity case, three inches long and two inches wide, with a chain handle. It contained powder, rouge, and lipstick, and was priced $18.

Chapter Three:
Carryalls

All types of compacts were made from the very plain to the very fancy, but the so-called "carryall" was probably the most popular of all. It was less expensive than the fancier minaudières and necessaires which made it more attractive to the average woman. And as the name implies, carryalls were arranged to carry all the items milady might want or need, yet they were not as bulky as a purse. A chain or mesh handle allowed them to be carried like a purse. The fancier ones and even the plainer ones were used more for parties and dates, while either could then be inserted into a case specially designed to turn the compact into a sort of dull purse. The cases that came with the carryalls were made of brocade, faille, suede, or any other suitable material. This variety in available materials proves that the competition was strong in the compact business and manufacturers were striving to please as many customers as possible—and please them it did, because the case allowed women to simply slip the carryall into it without having to transfer its contents to a purse and back again.

Although the carryall is generally rectangular in shape, there are a few square-shaped ones that have to be recognized as belonging in this category. As a general rule the square ones have less space or they might just have fewer items. But they always had a chain handle and most of them had a lipstick on the side. Of course other compacts had lipsticks on the side, but the handle seems to be the determining factor—with a handle it is a carryall, without one it is simply a compact. For most collectors the rectangular carryall is the pick of the litter. It was and is the most conveniently arranged, and has all the things anyone could need. Again it depends on the manufacturer and the style, but most carryalls have compartments for powder (either loose or pressed), rouge, lipstick, comb, and always a mirror. Some carryalls will have compartments for cigarettes, as most women smoked in those days, and some even have a built-in cigarette lighter. Some also have a place for money, both paper and coins, some with only a place for one while others have a place for both. This was one of the attractive features of the carryalls—they contained everything a woman could need, including money, so she could just slip it into its case and didn't have to move the contents to her purse and back again after a shopping trip. Since carryalls were a bit more expensive than regular compacts, chances are not as many of them were sold. The number available reflects this. And just as it was then, prices are much higher for carryalls than for the average compacts.

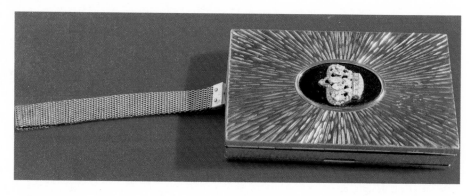

In 1949 this compact was advertised for $36.50. Made by Evans, it was described as the bracelet-handled Coronation Carryall fitted with after-five indespensables. $200-$250.

Inside this compact was a jeweler-designed automatic "pop-up" lipstick, according to one ad, and a covered powder well, puff, comb, and coin holder with the back designed for cigarettes. The space between the lipstick and powder originally had a fabric purse-like container for paper money, handkerchief, or keys.

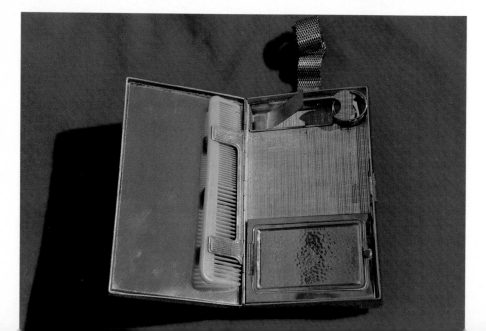

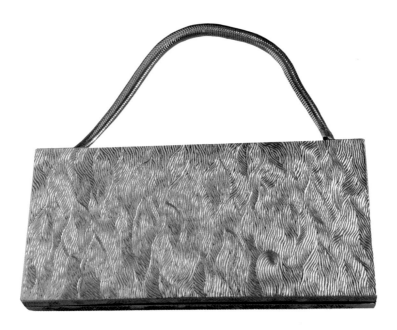

Silver metal carryall made by Evans. Handle is on the side rather than on the end. Pretty over-all design, snake chain. $150-$175.

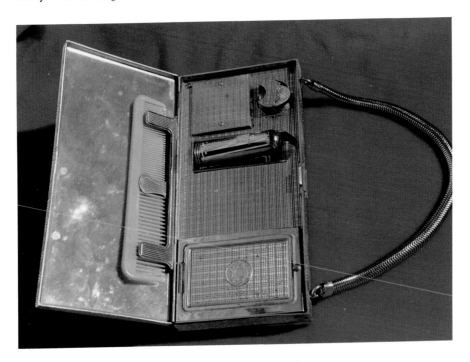

Inside very similar to Coronation carryall except this one also has a place for a lighter in the cigarette compartment. Both sides open.

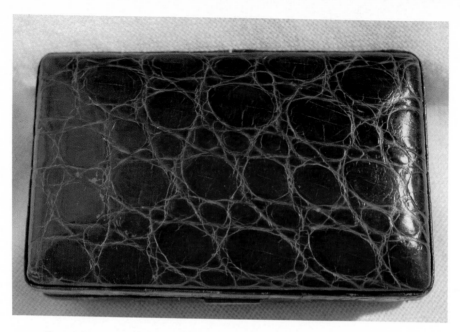

Small (2.5 by 4.5 inch) brown alligator carryall. Circa 1953. So well-designed it has everything the large carryalls have, including space for cigarettes in the domed top. Made by Elgin American. $150-$200.

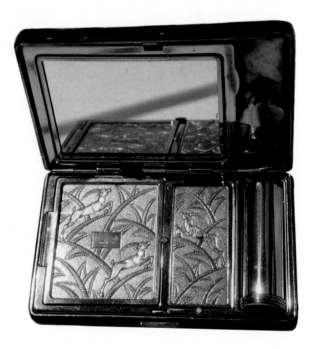

Inside has beautiful etched designs of leaping gazelles.

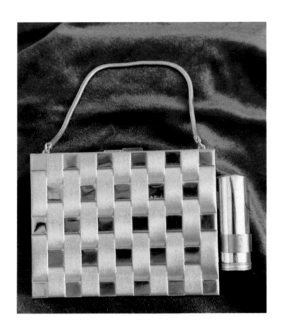

Goldtone glossy and matte basket weave carryall with lipstick on side. Only mark is Made in U. S. A. $50-$75.

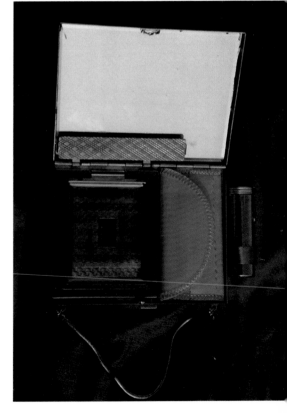

It is unusual now to find the fabric containers that could be used for paper money or keys that were standard with carryalls and compacts when they were new.

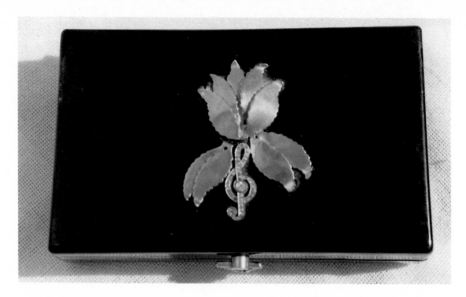

Imitation tortoise shell carryall, goldtone leaf design on top with rhinestone encrusted musical note. Appears to have never been used. Made by Henri Bendel, New York. $50-$75.

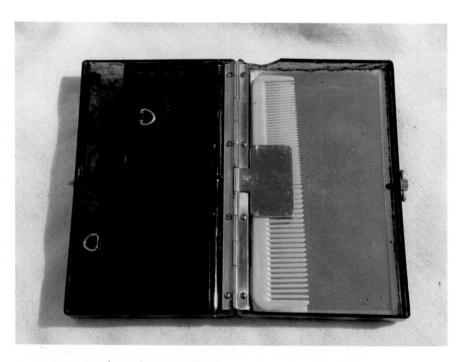

Powder and rouge wells have goldtone rings for opening.

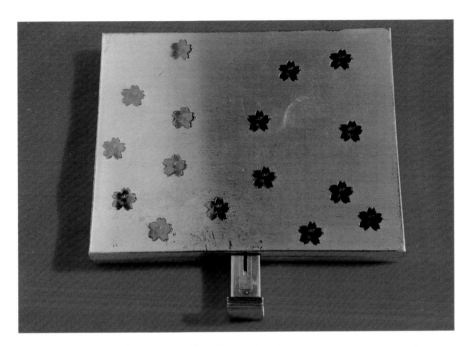

Large (5 by 6 inch), heavy carryall. Silver with goldtone decorations. Lipstick holder forms fastener. Maker unknown. Another one that seems to have seen little or no use. $75-$95.

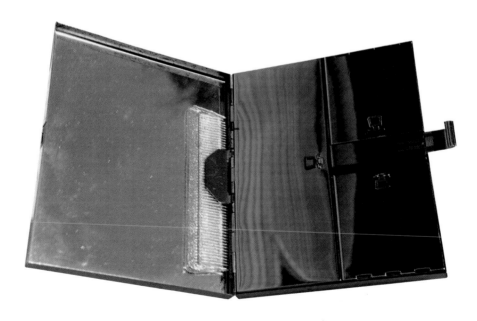

One opening, two wells in front while long back one is divided under the cover, perhaps for cigarettes and a lighter.

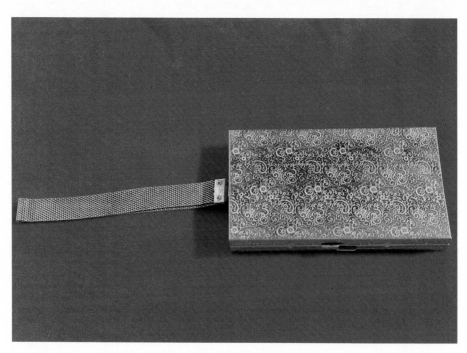

Goldtone, all-over design carryall. Mesh handle. Maker unknown. $85-$100.

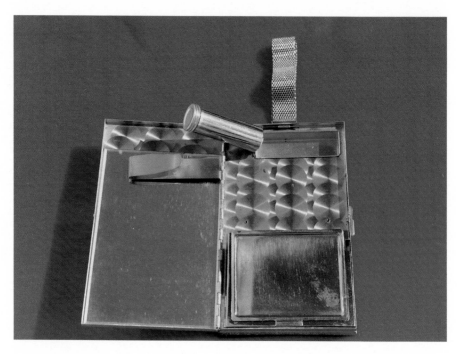

Automatic "pop-up" lipstick, both sides open, back is cigarette case.

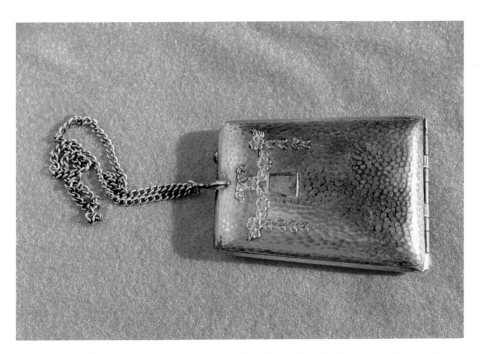

Art Deco designed silver purse or carryall. Likely identified as purse when made. Unusual placement of mirror over the powder well. Maker unknown. $60-$85.

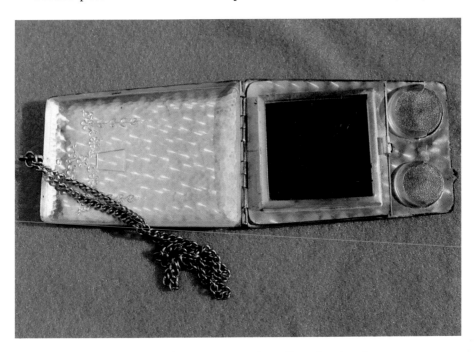

This compact has only a mirror, powder well, and a place for coins.

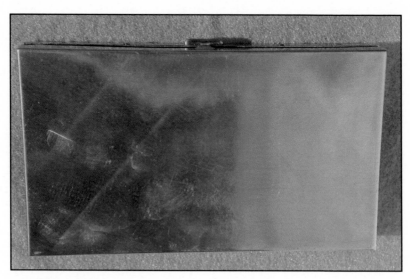

Plain goldtone carryall, no handle. Maker unknown. Due to the damage to the mirror it is not too desirable. $25-$35.

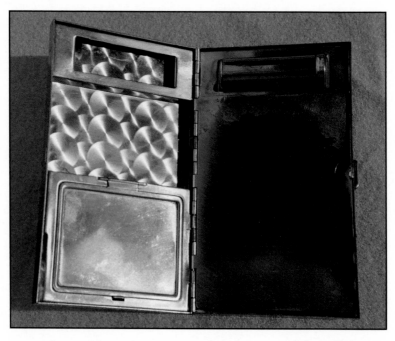

Mirror is damaged from what appears to have been something spilled on it.

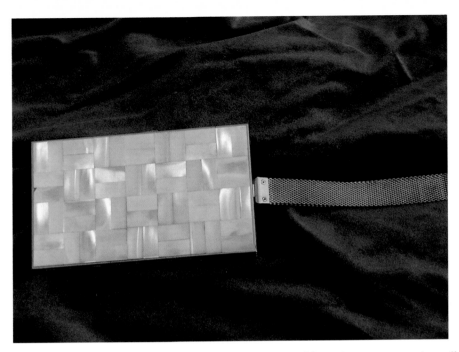

Mother-of-pearl on both sides of this carryall. Comb and lipstick missing, powder well appears to have never been used, yet the "Genuine Mother-of-Pearl by Anisco" label is still on the powder well. Mesh handle. $175-$225.

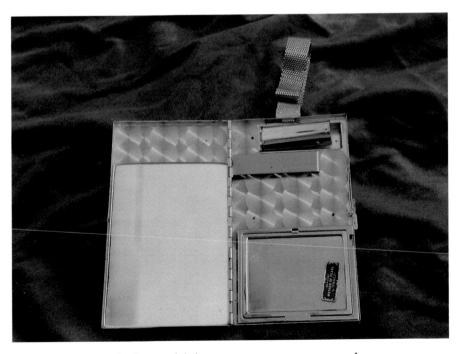

Inside showing label. Has cigarette case on one side.

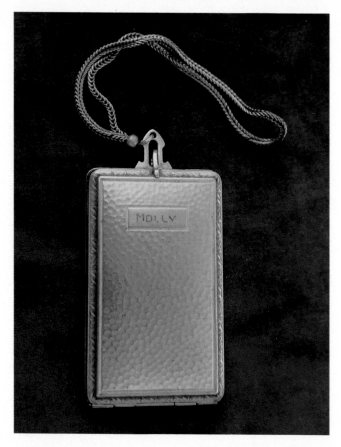

Many carryalls and compacts came with a place for a name or initials. The monogramming might be done in the store or by an engraver. Some of the less expensive ones came from the manufacturer with the most common girl's names already on them. Small carryall, approximately 2 by 3.5 inches. Maker unknown $45-$65.

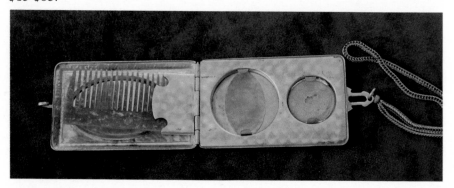

This carryall may be small but it has a mirror, powder and rouge wells, and a comb.

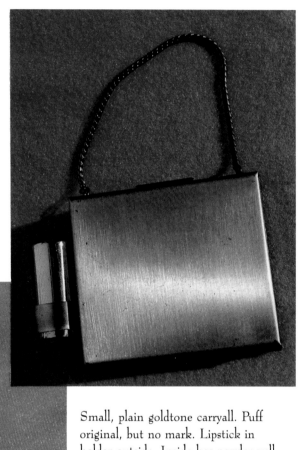

Small, plain goldtone carryall. Puff original, but no mark. Lipstick in holder outside. Inside has powder well and place for cigarettes. Inexpensive and unmarked. $25-$35.

Small carryall, imitation leather with factory embossed initial. Has never been used, but this is not that unusual as popular girls might receive as many as a dozen compacts and carryalls a year. She naturally used her favorites while others remained packed in drawers. If she didn't smoke, she might use the cigarette cases, especially on the small ones, for money or keys. Still in the original gift box. $45-$55.

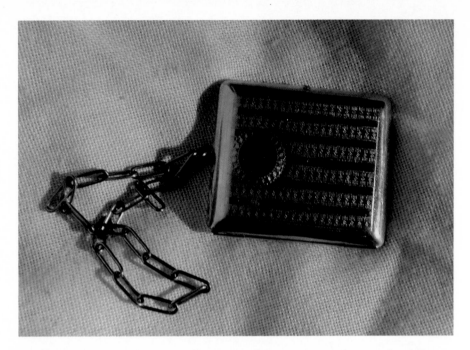

Small (2.25 by 2.5 inches) carryall, unmarked, but appears to be French-made. Unusual feature is the beveled mirror. Seldom seen in compacts or carryalls. $50-$75.

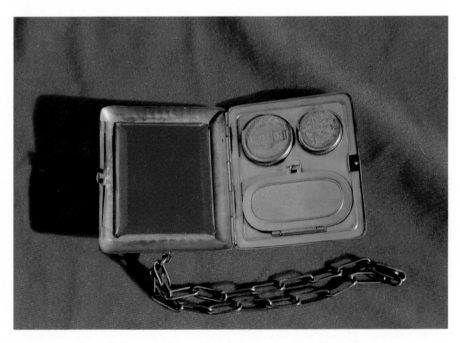

Inside only has powder well and slots for two different size coins.

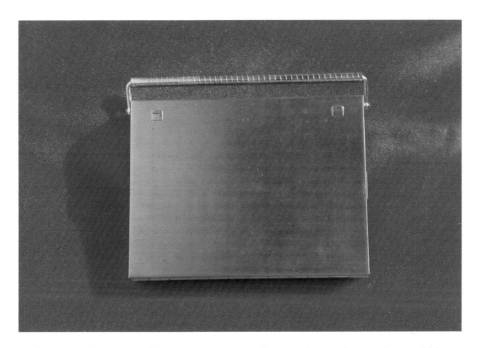

Volupté goldtone carryall. Unusual feature is decorated lipstick case that could have been added later. An identical carryall, except .5 an inch thicker to accommodate a cigarette case behind the mirror, was also made and came with a black faille carrying case. Roll handle. $100-$135.

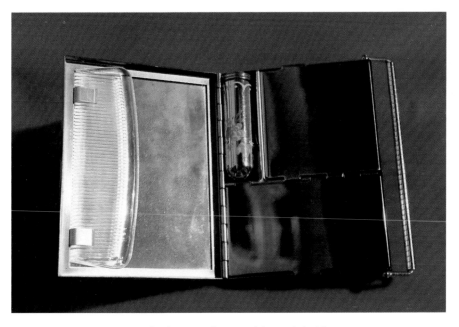

Inside showing decorated lipstick holder.

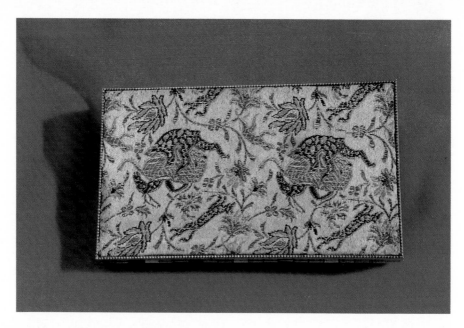

Persian scene, fabric covered carryall that is quite similar to the metal carryalls made by Volupté. Unmarked $100-$125.

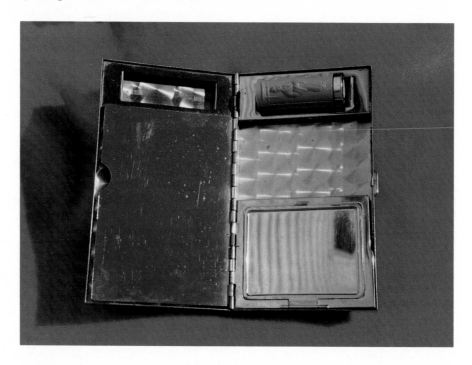

Inside very similar to other carryalls. Mirror is pulled down to reach the cigarette case.

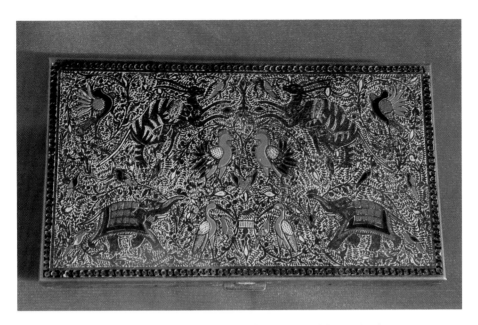

Brass with Persian enameled design. Still has fabric purse-like holder for money or comb. Pull down mirror reveals cigarette case. Volupté carryall. $125-$150.

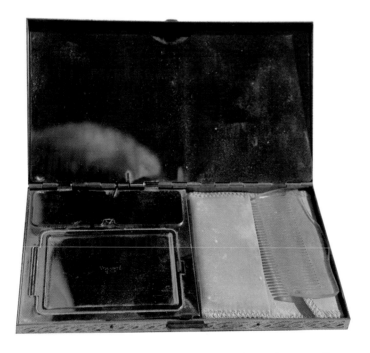

Comb shows how short they had to be to fit in the carryall.

Chapter Four:
Combinations—
Powder, Paint, and Lipstick

As we have already discussed, powder and paint has been through many ups and downs through the years. During the first quarter of the present century makeup was making a slow comeback. Women had been using powder—just to take the shine off their noses—for some time, and they had been known to pinch their cheeks to add a little color, but the thought of using store-bought rouge was just too much to comprehend. Naturally the majority of compacts were made with powder only. This was fine for married women, who did not dare paint their faces, but there were young girls, some who would become the Flappers of the Roaring twenties, who wanted both powder and paint. As usual the manufacturers were very aware of the wants and needs of their customers. They began making compacts that contained both powder and rouge. The surprising thing about this was they were able to make the same small compacts, some even smaller and thinner than the regular ones, and still include rouge. Some of the small compacts might even have two small rouge compartments, each with a different shade.

In the thirties and forties many young women used lipstick for both their lips and cheeks. They said they wanted the colors on both to match perfectly, and the only way to get it was to use lipstick on both. There was not a lot of difference in the lipstick and paste rouge so it worked perfectly. Probably with that thought in mind some compacts were made with two lipsticks—one on either side of the compact. Later small sized compacts would be made with powder, rouge, paste lipstick, and eye makeup, all in one compact. One of the things that makes compacts so intriguing is the variety. You never know what you are going to find, nor how it will be arranged inside.

Not everyone wanted a carryall or a compact with several compartments, they wanted individual containers of powder, rough and lipstick. Again the manufacturers were ready for the customers. They already had the simple powder compacts and then they made small, plain compacts of rouge only. Some of the lipsticks were put in elegant cases while others were encased in the plainest of cases. But for the customer who might want a plain lipstick but an elegant case, they made lipstick cases that could be used over and over to hold whatever lipstick the owner might buy.

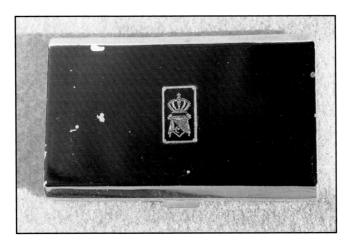

Small case (1.75 by 3 inches) holds a generous supply of cosmetics. One side has powder and rouge. Mirror can be pulled down to reveal paste lipstick, eye shadow, mascara, brush, and place for missing eyebrow pencil, Made by Zell. Black enameled case with use scars. Small crown design on top. $30-$50.

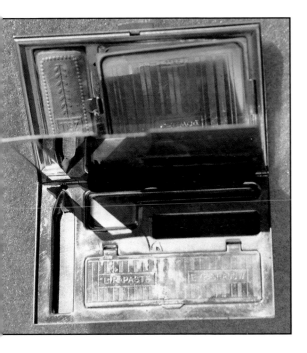

Showing well-arranged contents.

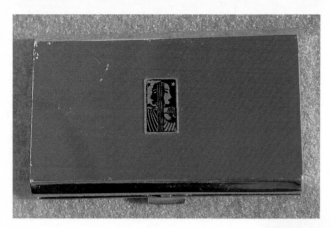

Compact identical in shape, size, and contents to the one above except case is red with design of woman's head instead of crown. Same cosmetics. Made by Zell. $30-$50.

Open compact showing contents.

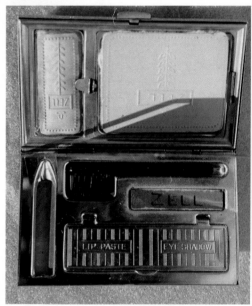

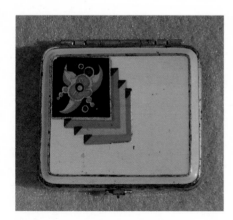

Small unmarked compact. Mirror separates powder and rouge—one on either side. $15-$22.

Pink enamel compact with silver trim. Loose powder well with sift thru. $18-$25.

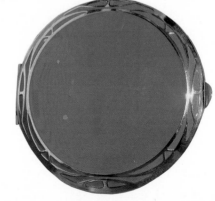

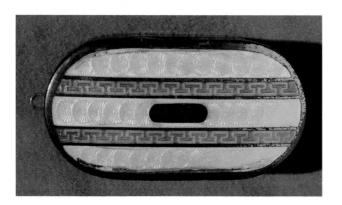

Pink and white Cloisonné case, small (1.5 by 2.5 inches), chain missing, mirror cracked. This is one of the reasons for buying damaged compacts, if the price is right. Parts like a handle from a badly damaged example could be used on this one. Unmarked. Damaged example $10-$12, perfect $35-$50.

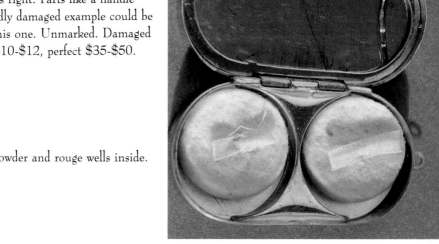

Has powder and rouge wells inside.

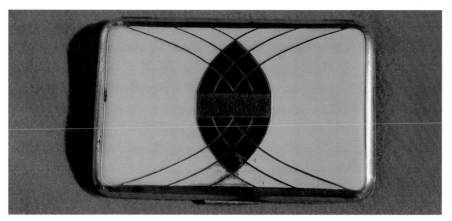

Richard Hudnut compact complete with powder, paint, and lipstick. $23-$35.

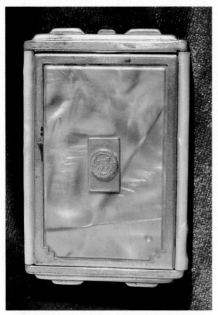

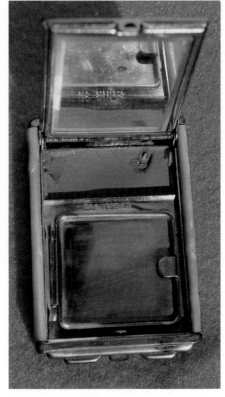

Souvenir compact from State Teachers College, Hyannis, Massachusetts. Made by Girey. Probably inexpensive originally, but surprisingly it has a beveled mirror. Top not cracked. $25-$35.

Has both powder and paint.

Puffs were usually marked with the maker's name.

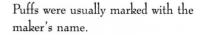

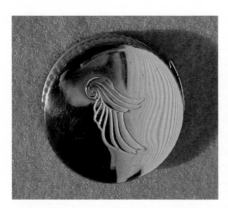

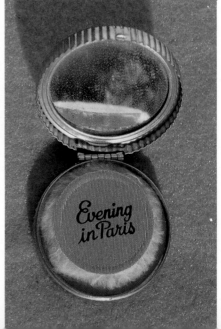

Individual compacts like this Evening in Paris rouge container could be carried in one's purse or left on the vanity. $10-$12.

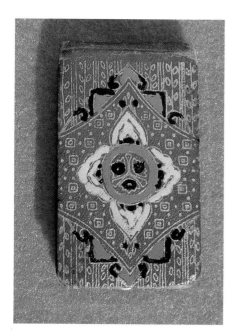

Imitation leather cover in bright colors. Small compact (1.5 by 2.75 inches) has well for pressed powder and rouge. Unmarked. $18 - $25.

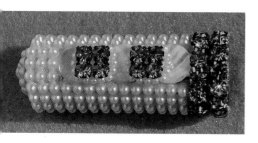

Lipstick case with amethyst stones set on mother-of-pearl design on the front and around the base. Balance of case covered in imitation pearls. Unmarked. $50-$75.

Some women didn't want a single compact or carryall with all their cosmetics, instead they wanted individual items like this tin of Pompeian Bloom pressed rouge. $10-$12.

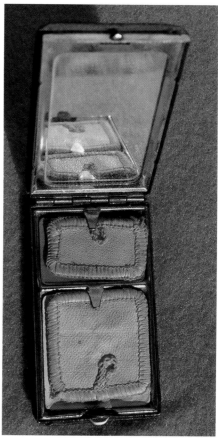

Vinyl covered puffs—white for powder, pink for rouge.

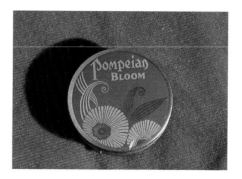

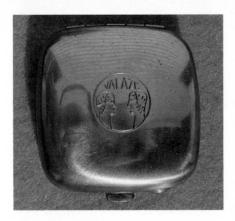

Square 1.75 inch, brass compact. Helena Rubenstein, New York, London, and Paris trademark. $27-$38.

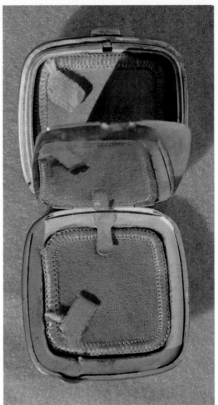

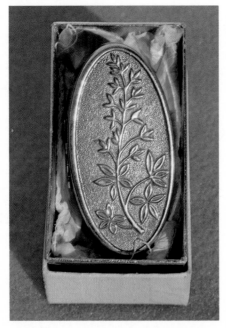

Small but with well-utilized space. Powder well on one side of mirror, rouge on the other.

When opened the case had a small mirror.

Max Factor lipstick case still in original box. When first purchased the price for this Golden Floral hi-society Red on Red lipstick was $2.50. Case only sold for $1.50, refill was $1. Also printed on the bottom was the information there was no Federal tax on the case. $25-$35.

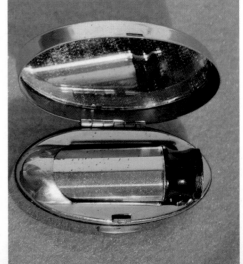

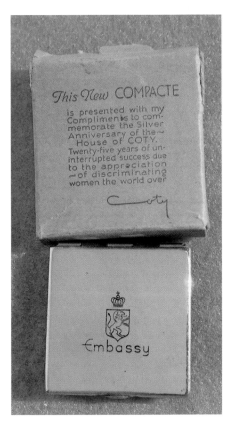

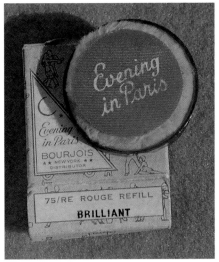

An Evening in Paris pressed rouge refill. This one, too, is probably worth more as advertising than as a cosmetic. $7-$10.

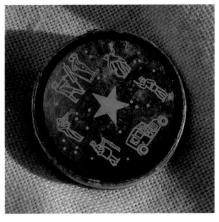

Cosmetic companies have always given lagniappes, a small gift of appreciation for their purchases, to customers. Coty gave this compact to customers on their silver anniversary, according to the information on the box. Embassy trademark on blue enameled top. Black bottom. Worth more now as an advertising piece than a compact. $20-$30.

Lagniappe from Evening in Paris. "Complimentary rouge" printed on the back confirms it. $5-$7.

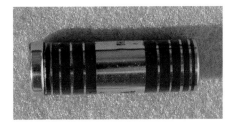

Park & Tilford lipstick in cases like this were staples in the ten cent stores during the thirties through the fifties. They could be bought then for 10 to 25 cents. $5-$8.

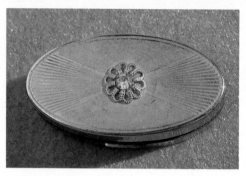

Max Factor lipstick designed a little differently. Style the same. $13-$18.

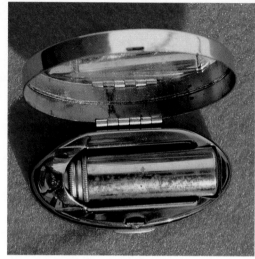

Color of lipstick in this case is Tangee Theatrical Red.

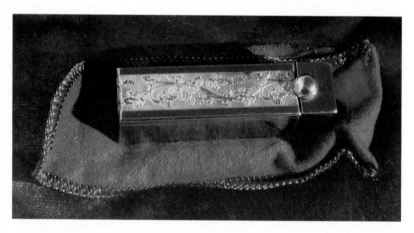

Volupté lipstick case still in original box. $25-$35.

Case open showing how mirror pops up as lipstick is removed.

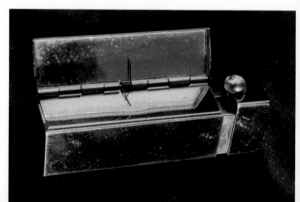

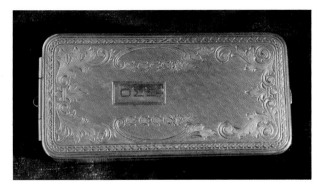

This compact looks like it was made of gold probably due to the Victorian design. Small (1.5 by 3.5 inches), mono-grammed, has powder, rouge, and lipstick. Originally had chain handle. Marked DuBarry, Richard Hudnut. With handle $45-$65, without $30-$50.

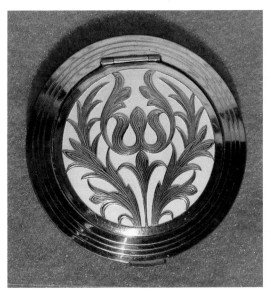

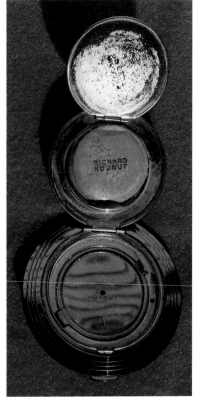

Richard Hudnut double foldout. Mirror folds over rouge, then both form a top that folds over the powder, and forms the top of the compact. $35-$50.

Same compact open.

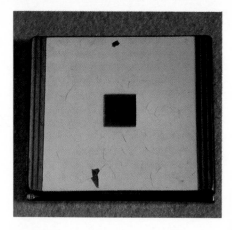

Metalfield compact, white enamel on goldtone. Never been used but enamel is chipping. $28-$39.

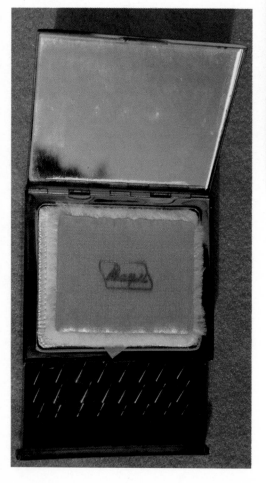

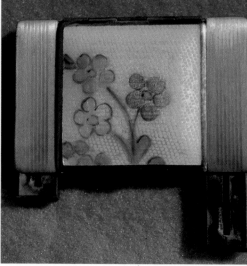

LaMode, small, well-arranged compact with floral Cloisonné design. Anna engraved on the back. $60-$85.

Thick case, bottom pulls out to form cigarette case. Nice satin puff.

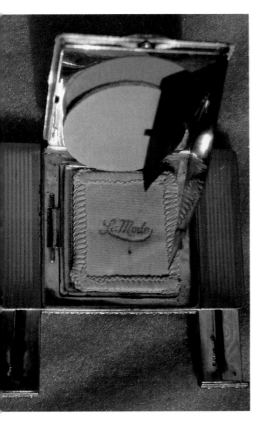

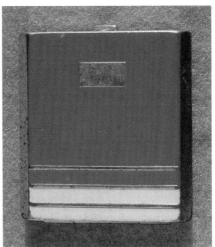

Small (2 inch square) Barbara Gould compact packed with cosmetics. Has pressed powder well, pop-up lipstick, and two places for pressed rouge. $35-$45.

Inside showing arrangement of powder, rouge, and lipstick tubes on either side.

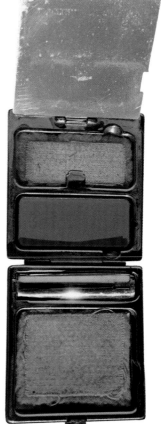

Inside showing arrangement of cosmetics.

Chapter Five:
Florals and Leaves

The decorations on compacts utilized just about every known design, but since they were made predominately for women the manufacturers seem to have leaned towards florals. Flowers, leaves, or both with an occasional butterfly appear to have been favorites. Such designs were applied on porcelain, metal, or fabric and seem to have become a favorite with the women. This opinion is based on the fact that so many compacts with those designs are available today. There are some with ordinary floral designs and then there are those with absolutely choice decorations.

One of these choice designs is shown here. It was made in Japan, using the Art of Chokin according to the label found inside it. The label reads that "The images are created by etching pure copper and then gilding it with silver and gold," and goes on to explain that this style of decoration is over 800 years old and was originally created to decorate the armament, especially the swords, of the Samurai warriors. According to the label found on another piece of this same type of work, it was originally introduced in the Sixth century to decorate shrines and temples and was used later on the Samurai swords and helmets. Whatever its origin, it is one of the most elegant designs we have seen. Late examples of this art, the Art of Chokin, have been found on powder boxes, small plates, jewelry boxes, and this one compact.

Some of these designs are applied, like the brass leaf on a metal compact, while others are handmade, as in the case of the petit point design. Incidentally, the bottom of the petit point design compact, along with several others with needlework tops, have a mesh bottom which is so light it is believed to be aluminum. The popularity of both the flowers and the leaves stems from its great variety. All types of flowers can be used, alone or with other blossoms, and leaves have the same appeal because of the many ways they can be used.

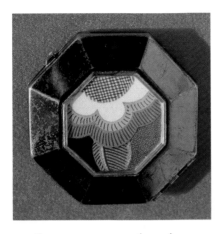

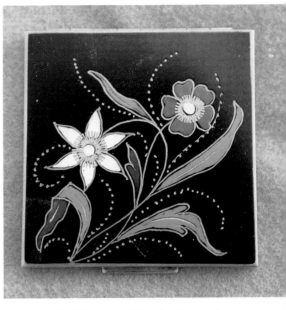

Small, inexpensive, powder only compact. $8-$10.

Enameled flower on black background, powder only, beveled mirror. Shields trademark. $35-$45.

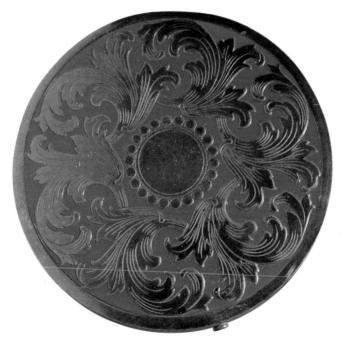

Large, flapjack-type compact, powder only. Other compacts made with the same decoration, but different colored background. Rex Fifth Avenue trademark. $30-$40.

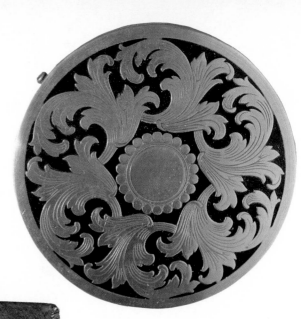

Rex Fifth Avenue flapjack with black background under leaf design. Original puff missing. $25-$40.

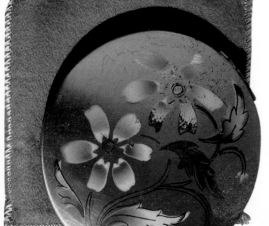

Round Dorset Fifth Avenue compact, powder only, blue flowers on goldtone base. $35-$45.

Goldtone, round, powder only compact with embossed, enameled flowers. Still in gift box. Puff marked Hampden. $40-$65.

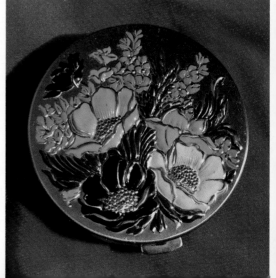

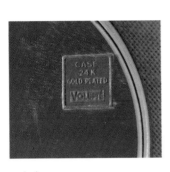

Label on mirror.

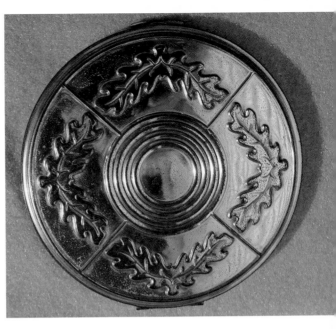

Large, round, powder only compact with leaf design. Label on mirror describes it as a 22 Karat gold plated case by Volupté. $150-$200.

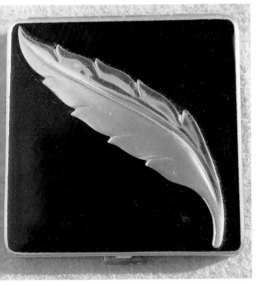

Half matte-half glossy goldtone leaf on black enamel background. Unmarked. $35-$50.

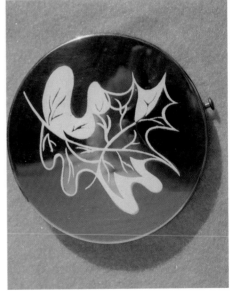

Large pink and gold leaf on red background. Powder only. Made by Columbia Fifth Avenue. $33-$45.

45

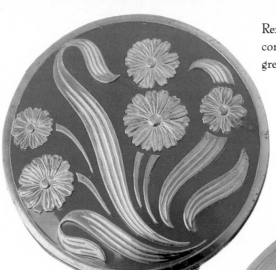

Rex Fifth Avenue flapjack-type powder compact. Goldtone floral decoration on green background. $28-$39.

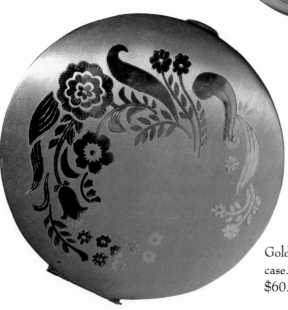

Goldtone case with cutout design of flower and butterfly on black background. Powder well cover same size as mirror. Marked Paris, made in France. $65-$85.

Goldtone floral design on goldtone case. Powder only. Unmarked. $40-$60.

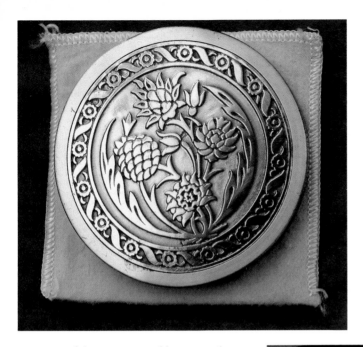

Beautiful Henriette, goldtone powder compact with original puff. Never been used. $50-$75.

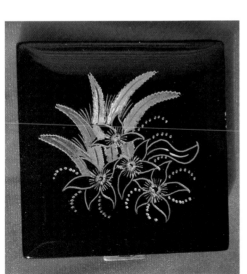

Powder only compact with Harriet Hubbard Ayers, Inc, New York trademark. $38-$46.

Both compact and puff are marked Majestic. Black enamel case with floral design in gold. $35-$50.

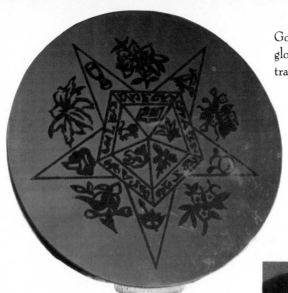

Goldtone powder only compact with glossy design. Columbia Fifth Avenue trademark. $45-$60.

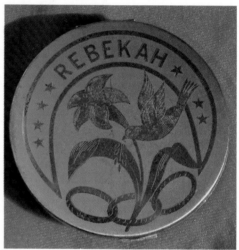

Goldtone flower and bird design for Rebekahs, Elgin American trademark. $50-$75

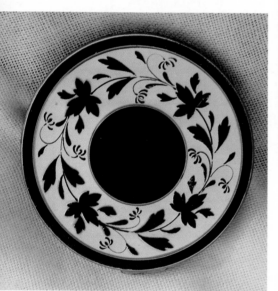

Raised black leaves on white ground, powder only, unmarked. $25-$37.

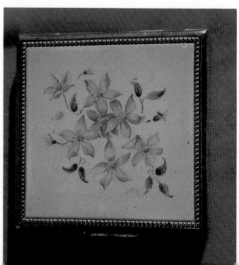

Square, Evans powder compact, pastel floral design, $20-$30.

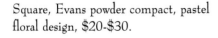

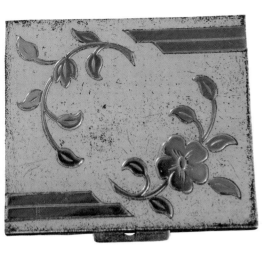

A questionable acquisition. The inside is perfect and lovely, but the outside has seen a lot of wear and tear, however judging by the inside there was not much use. Ritz trademark. If price is right, would make a good compact for everyday use or mirror might fit an otherwise expensive compact without one. Fair price for this one is $7-$9.

Close-up showing design in more detail.

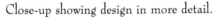

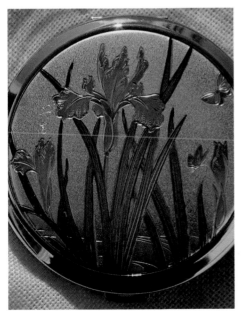

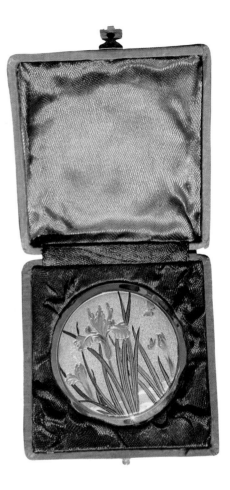

Compact decorated with the Art of Chokin originally used in the 6th century to decorate shrines and temples. Later it would be used on Samurai armor, swords, and helmets. In recent years it has been used on compacts, powder boxes, and musical jewelry boxes. The compact was made in Japan for the Westland Company who distributed it under the trade name Lovely. The process is created by etching copper plate and gilding it with gold and silver. In gift box. $200-$250.

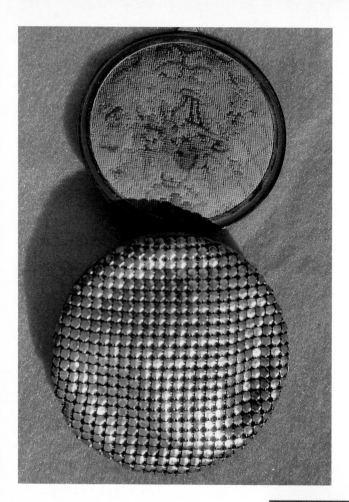

Imported petit point in top, link mesh
bottom (could be aluminum), powder in
bottom, rouge under mirror. Evans.
$60-$85.

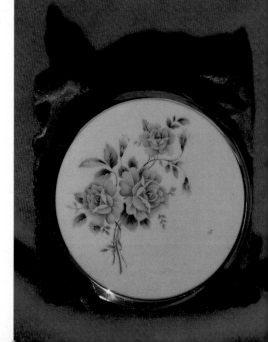

Another compact that has never been
used. Made by Stratton of England.
$25-$35.

Chapter Six:
Goldtones

Indications are that the majority of gold colored compacts were made later, around the forties and fifties. This is based on researching several older wholesale jeweler's catalogs. One 1932 catalog with ten pages of compacts only listed half a dozen with a finish other than an enameled, non-tarnishing chromium finish. These illustrations not only showed the various designs, but listed the enamel colors. Incidentally, most of the colors were dark like black, brown, blue, and green. Very few were listed with a white enameling, several had black and white while less than half a dozen used any pastel colors. Three were listed with a "green gold finish" while a few had sterling silver tops. Several pages of compacts were shown in color, but not one was described as goldtone or gold colored.

Although the goldtones, also called gold colored and jeweler's bronze, seem to be more plentiful now than any other color, apparently they were made later. This can be confirmed by their style and decorations. One would probably have to have a degree in metallurgy to be able to identify the metals in most of the compacts today. It is easy to identify the ones marked sterling silver or gold plated. Then there are a few solid gold ones, but the average collector isn't apt to find one of those. Most of us know brass when we see it, but some of the compacts found today seem to be made of alloys.

It is doubtful the average compact collector today really cares what material was used to make the compact unless it was pure gold or silver. They are more interested in the style, the decoration, the compartments, and the shape. If they plan to use it, shape and size would be important. A large compact will not fit into some of the small purses being used today. Condition is also important when buying a compact, whether to use or to add to one's collection. If the price is right, a slightly damaged compact would be satisfactory for daily use, but if it was going into a collection, the collector should look for one in as nearly perfect condition as possible. The logic here is that one used daily will eventually show wear and tear anyway, so it isn't that important it be absolutely perfect in the beginning. On the other hand collections are generally assembled as an investment; therefore it behooves the collectors to buy the most perfect examples available.

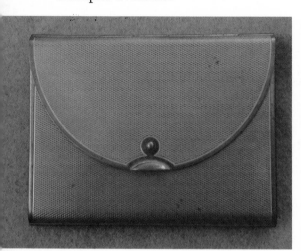

Unusual-shaped Coty compact which opens like an envelope. $85-$100.

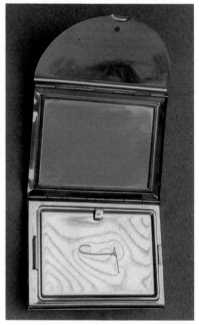

Coty compact open.

American made compact with trapeze artists design. $40-$60.

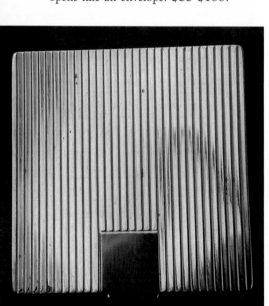

Square goldtone Coty. $50-$70.

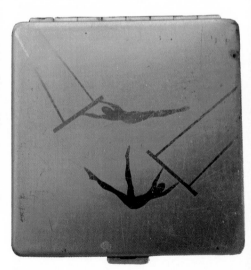

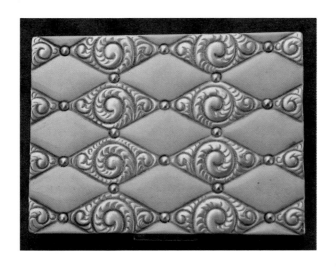

Ivory celluloid with goldtone design. Unmarked. $40-$50.

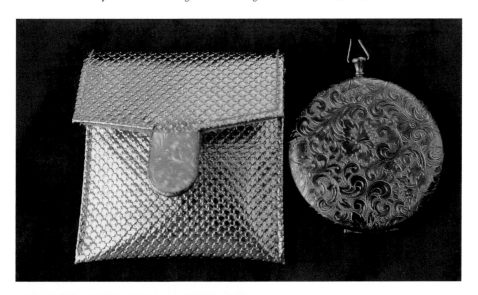

Zell compact shaped like a pocket watch in goldtone case. $60-$85.

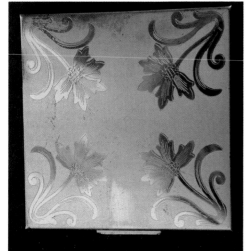

Elgin American with glossy goldtone design. $45-$75.

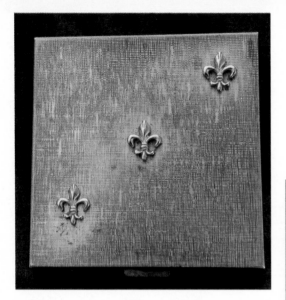

Volupté compact, goldtone with fleur-de-lis design. $50-$75.

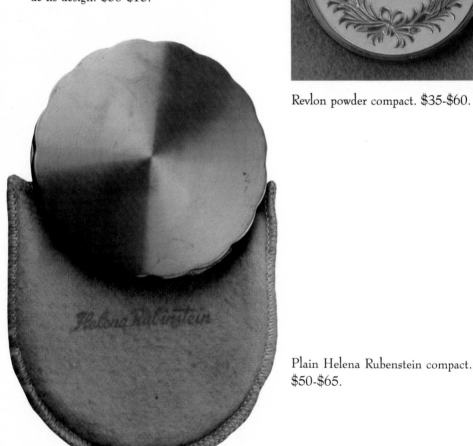

Revlon powder compact. $35-$60.

Plain Helena Rubenstein compact. $50-$65.

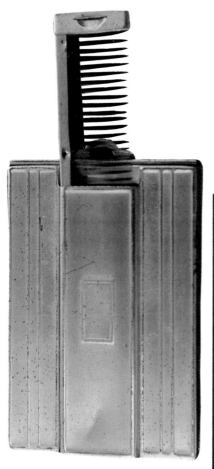

Oblong powder compact with comb in the top, beveled mirror, K & K trademark. $60-$80.

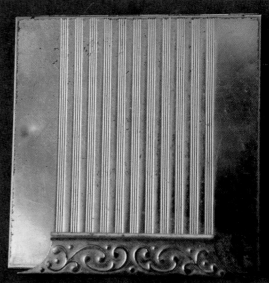

Front clasp pulls down to open, Avon. $25-$35.

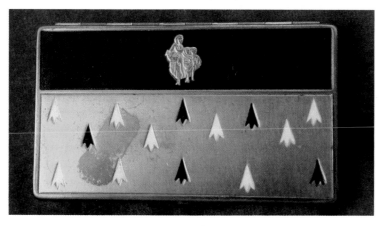

Black and goldtone Yardley powder and rouge compact. $45-$55.

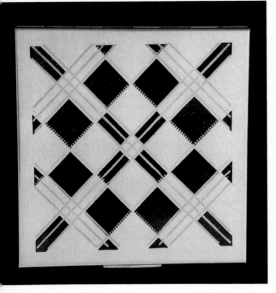

Zell goldtone with black enamel design. $40-$55.

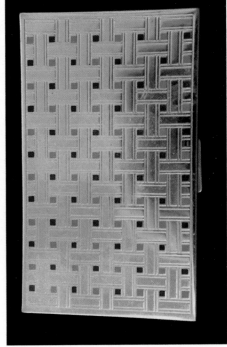

Richard Hudnut compact with red and black enameled dots. $45-$70.

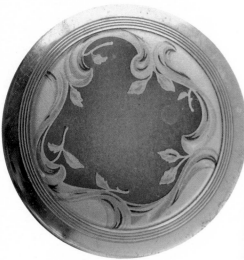

Coty pressed powder compact. $35-$45.

Volupté compact with rhinestone fastener. $40-$50.

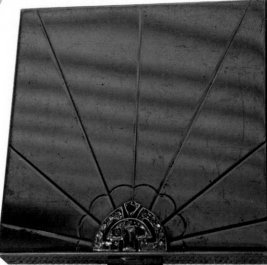

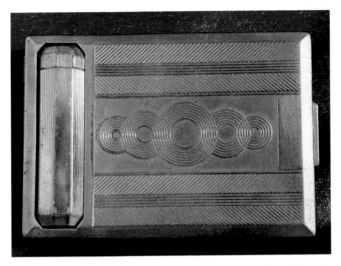

Powder, rouge, and lipstick compact by Richard Hudnut. $75-$90.

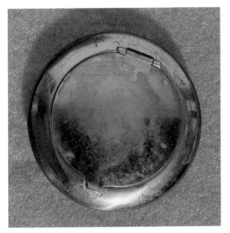

Small compact looks like it was made of brass, unmarked. $15-$20.

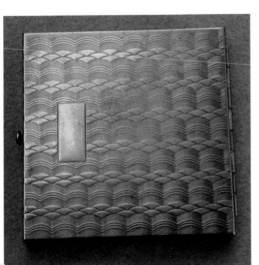

Showing the inside of the compact.

Goldtone compact with place for monogram. $30-$40.

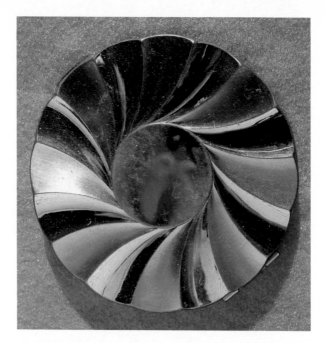

Powder only compact by Majestic. $25-$35.

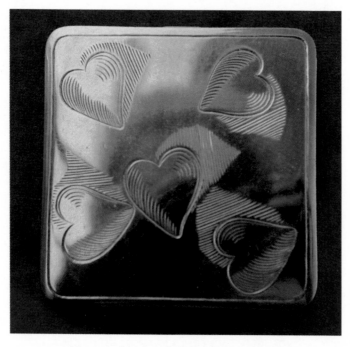

Goldtone compact with heart design. $30-$40.

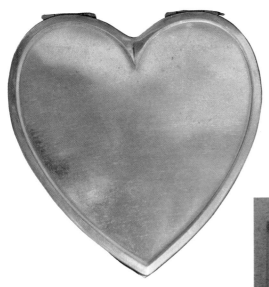

Heart-shaped compact, Superb trademark. $55-$70.

Clear Lucite base with round goldtone compact on top. Made by Belle. $50-$65.

Quality compact with design on both sides, beveled mirror, unmarked. $50-$65.

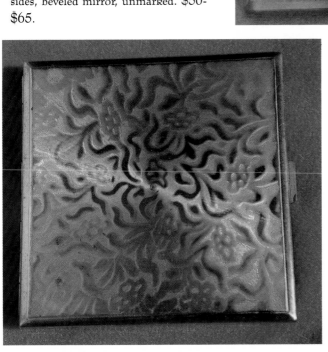

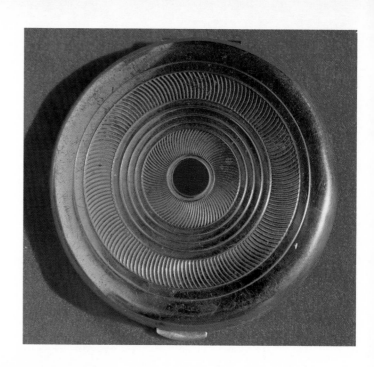

Coty compact with Air Spun powder. $30-$40.

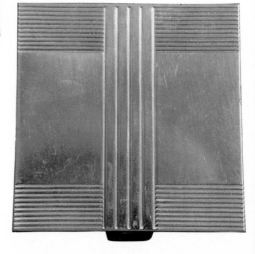

Compact with sword and crown decoration. $38-$65.

Plain compact by Volupté. $42-$58.

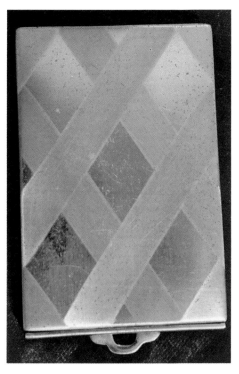

Powder compact made by K & K. $35-$60.

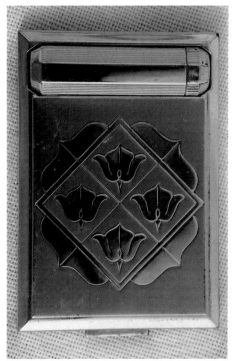

Powder, rouge, and lipstick compact by Richard Hudnut. $65-$78.

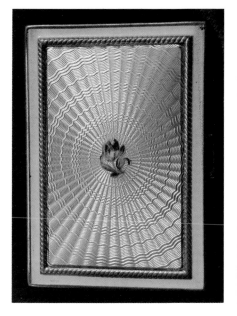

Rex compact, powder and rouge, Cloisonné top. $68-$75.

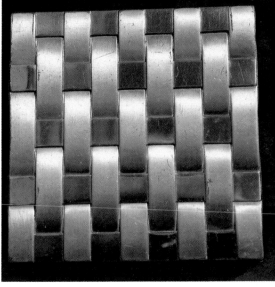

Goldtone, basketweave compact by Evans. $65-$80.

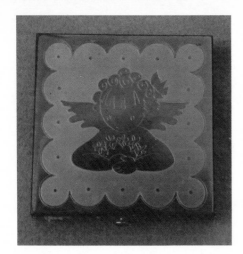

Angel/child design by Wadsworth. $25-$38.

Rex compact with bow design on top. $35-$45.

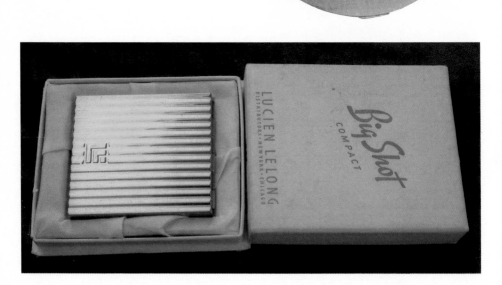

Lucien LeLong's Big Shot compact in original box. $75-$90.

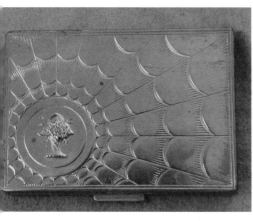

Cara Nome powder and rouge compact. $35-$50.

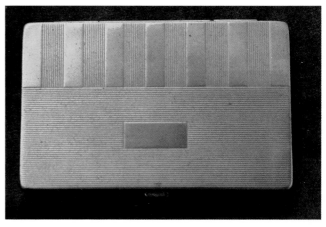

Elgin American compact. $50-$70.

Houbigant powder and rouge compact, place for monogram. $35-$45.

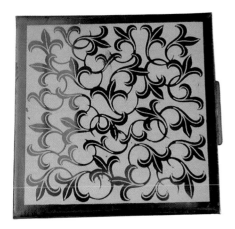

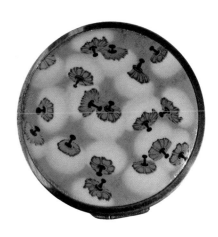

Powder puff design seems to have been a trademark for Coty. $40-$65.

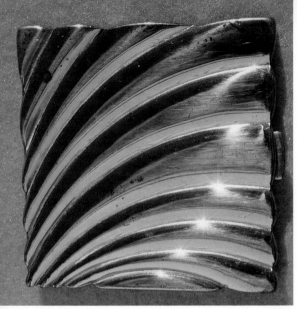

Heavy Volupté powder compact. $40-$65.

Fianceé Woodworth powder and rouge compact. $45-$55.

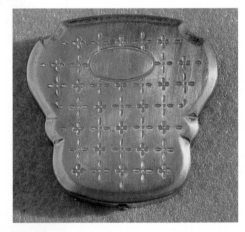

Cara Nome (Langlois, Boston) powder compact. $35-$50.

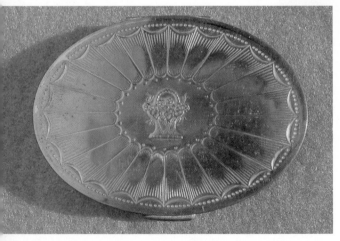

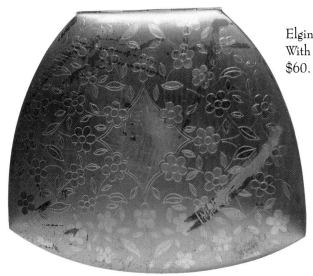

Elgin American goldtone compact. With damage $15-$20, perfect $40-$60.

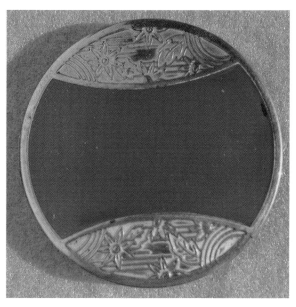

Vashé powder and rouge compact. $50-70.

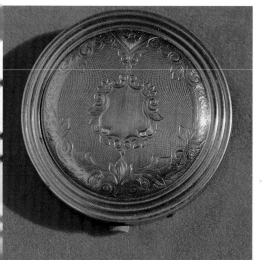

Zell powder compact, resembles pocket watch. $50-$65.

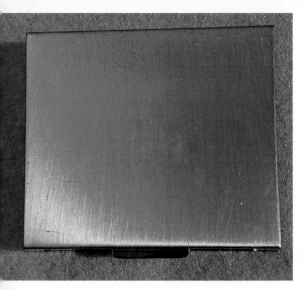

Plain, unmarked compact. $25-$35.

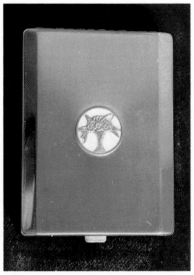

Small Cara Nome powder compact. $25-$35.

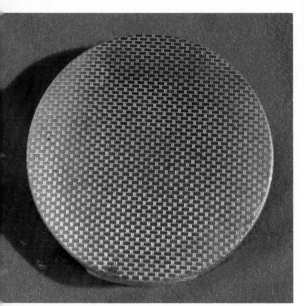

Gigi pressed powder compact. $25-$35.

66

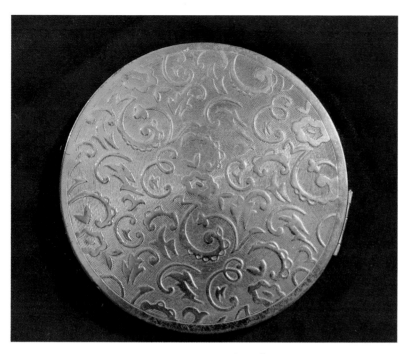

Large Rex compact. $40-$60.

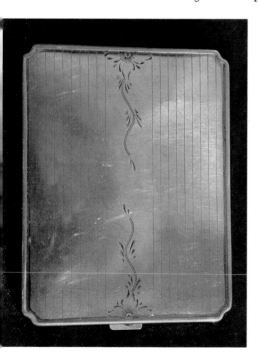

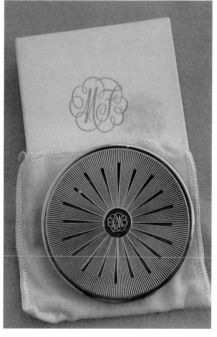

Unmarked powder and rouge compact.
$40-$55.

Max Factor Creme Puff compact in
original box. $60-$75.

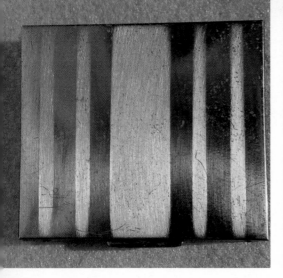

Inexpensive, unmarked compact. $15-$20.

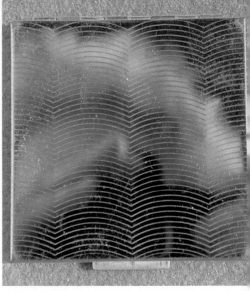

Rex Fifth Avenue compact. $35-$45.

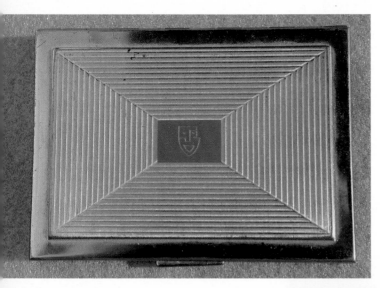

Max Factor powder and rouge compact. $50-$70.

Elizabeth Arden powder compact, never used. $50-$65.

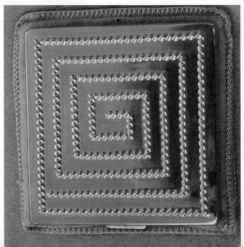

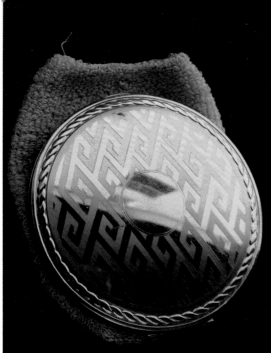

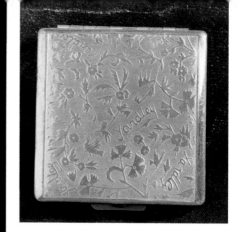

Small Yardley compact. $35-$45.

Elgin American flapjack. $70-$85.

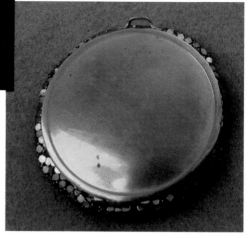

Volupté compact, design on both sides. $45-$65.

Solid brass top, mesh bottom. $45-$60

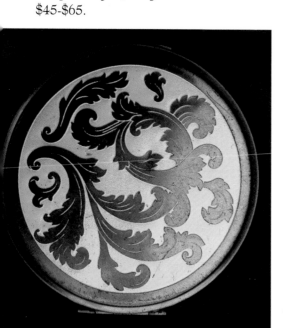

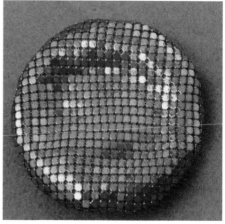

Mesh bottom

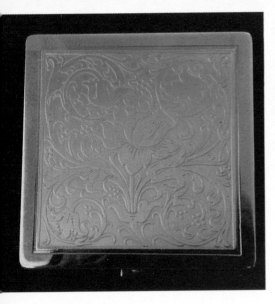

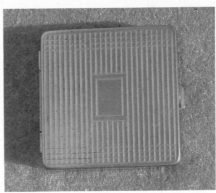

Goldtone 1.5 inch square powder compact, Elizabeth Arden name in three places—on the bottom, puff, and pressed powder. $25-$30.

Easterling, well-made compact. $50-$75.

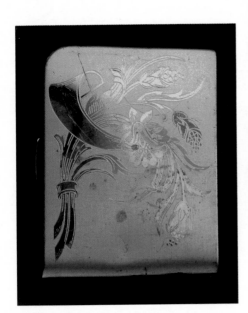

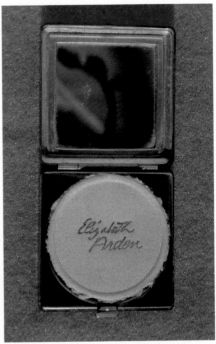

Inside showing name on puff.

Elgin American with floral design. $50-$65.

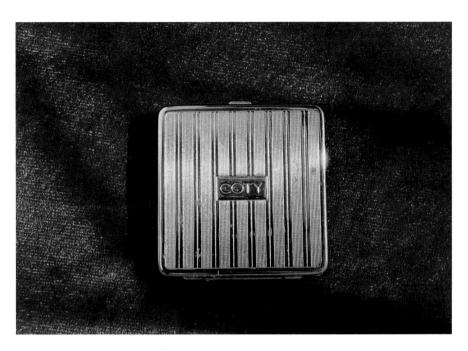

Goldtone Coty compact. $25-$35.

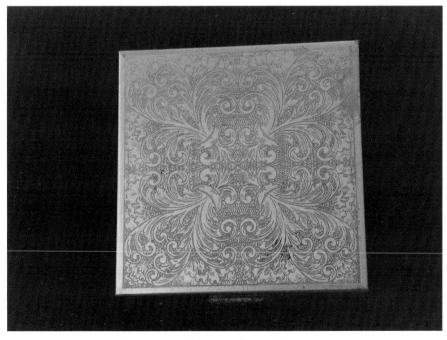

Large Rex with ornate design. $50-$75.

Chapter Seven:
Jeweled Tops

Variety is one of the reasons compacts have always been so popular. The materials used to make them are as varied as their shapes and sizes, but most importantly, it seems, is the design or decoration on the top. They can range from etched decorations to jewels, imitation stones and pearls to be sure, but jewels nevertheless. Some of the very expensive compacts, those made for wealthy customers, had the real thing in both gold and sterling cases as well as precious and semi-precious stones. But the majority of compacts found by collectors today will have imitation pearls and stones. Some of these, however, are very attractive. Like everything else some are better than others.

One of the compacts pictured here has a small jade design on a plain, goldtone compact. The green against the gold is most attractive. Another has a round decorated top on a square compact. The round top has two rows of white glass stones resembling rhinestones around a circle of the same stones separated by two narrow rows of lattice-type goldtone metal set with small white glass stones at rather spaced intervals. The overall effect is very eye catching. A small, goldtone compact has a bunch of grapes with leaves on the top. Again, it is difficult to identify the metal without some kind of mark, yet the bunch of grapes looks suspiciously like it might be made of sterling.

Another attractive compact is one made of a gold colored metal with a branch of what looks like mistletoe. The white mistletoe berries are made of imitation pearls. Another compact has row after row of imitation pearls covering the top. Another example that is very attractive is a goldtone compact with a V made of blue glass stones in various sizes, starting with small ones on the top and ending with a large one on the bottom. The majority of the jeweled top compacts are gold colored, but there are exceptions. For instance, a square, black enameled one has two gold lines across the top and bottom and down either side of a small square with a basket of bejeweled flowers in the center. Another interesting compact is a narrow width Prince Matchabelli in copper with black enameling. Just a narrow line of the copper shows around the edge of the top and bottom with another line down either side with his trademark, a fancy crown, in raised copper in the center. This compact might not be jeweled, but it still has a crown.

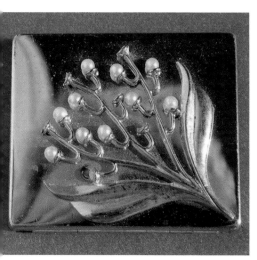

Excellent compact for use at Christmas as sprig of imitation pearls looks like mistletoe. Made by Flato. $25-$40.

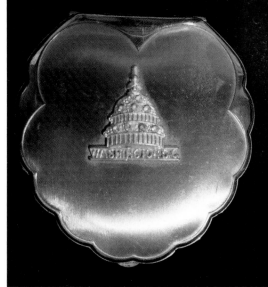

Souvenir Washington, D.C. compact. Jeweled windows in capitol, Elgin American trademark. $60-$75.

Fancy compact with a lipstick on either side, large jeweled design on top. Made by Majestic. $60-$75.

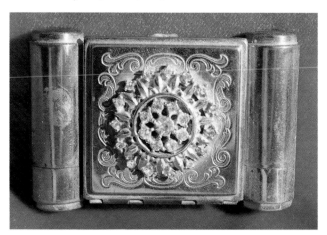

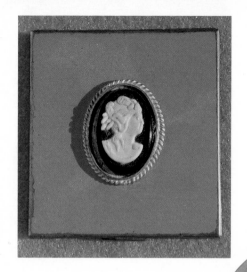

Not exactly jeweled but has nice cameo on top. Foster trademark. $30-$40.

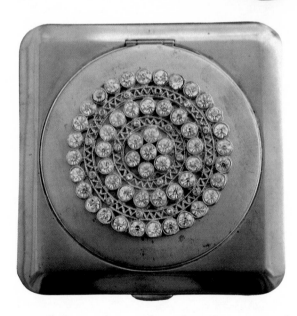

Oval-shaped compact with jeweled floral design. $30-$40.

Ornately decorated top, only mark Made in U.S.A. $65-$75.

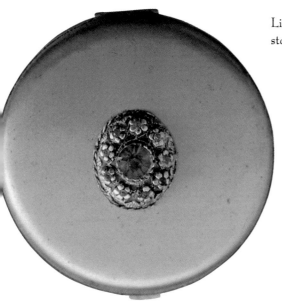

Lin Bren compact with colored glass stones on top. $40-$50.

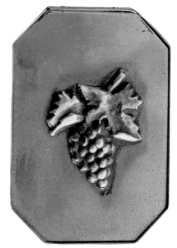

Unusual-shaped compact. To open hinge cover has to be pulled down and pressure exerted on back of compact cover. Unmarked. $45-$50.

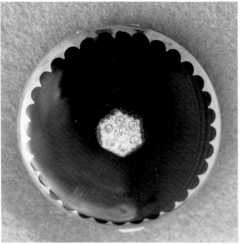

Black top with scalloped goldtone border, small jewel on top. Unmarked. $30-$40.

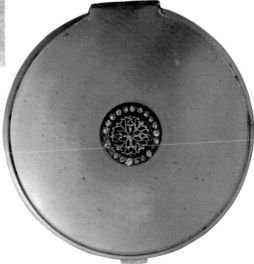

Rouge compartment is recessed into powder well. Unmarked. $40-$50.

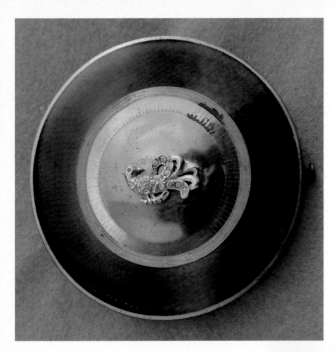

Large compact, powder only, jeweled bird on cover. Columbia. $45-$60.

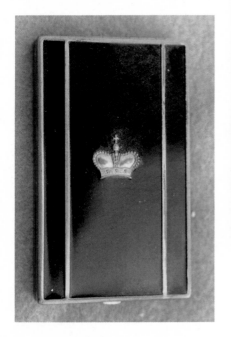

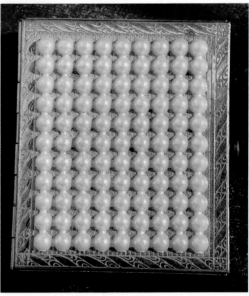

Dorset compact, top covered with imitation pearls. $35-$50.

Prince Matchabelli compact, crown on top. $50-$65.

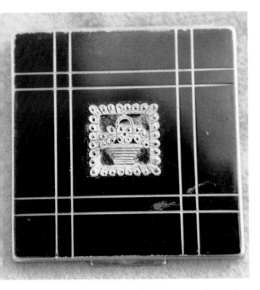

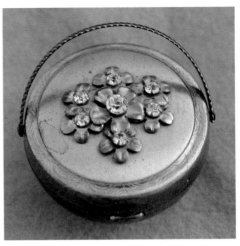

Shields compact with marcasite framed basket of flowers on top. $50-$60.

A 1.5 inch tall basket-shaped compact. $85-$95.

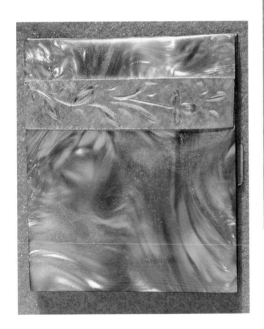

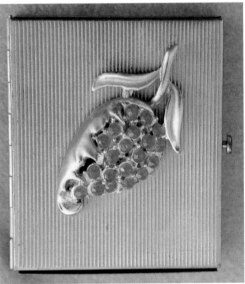

Dorset compact, leaf filled with red glass stones on top. $30-$45.

Etched band looks like jewels. Unmarked. $45-$65.

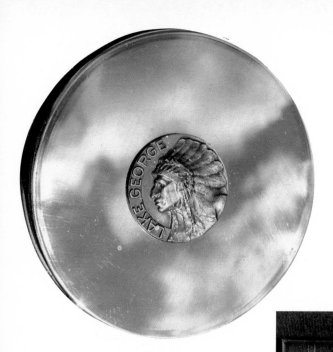

Rex compact. Indian head decoration. Souvenir from Lake George (New York). $50-$65.

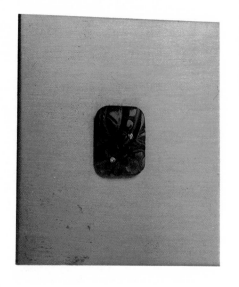

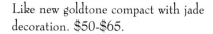

Volupté compact with V set in blue glass stones. $25-$35.

Like new goldtone compact with jade decoration. $50-$65.

Chapter Eight:
Leather and Fabric Covers

Few compacts were made that cannot be classified in two or more categories. About the only exceptions are a few of the plain fabric or leather covered varieties. Ones that might pass for a simple fabric-covered compact could have designs, either printed, or in some type of needlework. Some of the leather ones are studded or monogrammed. As we have said before the variety of compacts that were made during their heyday is overwhelming. Manufacturers were trying desperately to corner their share of the market which explains why they designed and made so many styles. If they made enough, they must have reasoned, surely there would be a style that fit everybody's idea of the perfect compact. And that is what makes compact collecting so intriguing today—you never know what you are going to find at the next show or the next mall.

You might find a leather covered compact, a plain one, or one with a monogram. Or you might get lucky and find one made of alligator or reptile. A cheaper leather version is the ornately decorated example which appears to have been made in India or after the colorful Indian style of decorating leather. This one has no mark or identification; therefore it is impossible to establish its maker. In this one the puff that might have had the name of the maker is missing. Of course collectors can not always rely on the name on the puff as it is not always the original one. A dirty puff was considered a disgrace in those days so the women often bought new puffs to replace the soiled ones. The puffs might have the name of their maker, or they might not have a name at all, but it wasn't often that puffs were replaced with ones like the original. Then there might be several girls in the family, all with half a dozen compacts each. And as girls have always done they would swap and trade—the puff from this compact for the one in another. It was ever thus. And that explains why you can't identify a compact by the puff alone, you must have other proof.

Often it is next to impossible to classify fabric covered compacts, that is, to determine if they are some type of brocade fabric or petit point. On some, like one from Evans, it is extremely easy because there is a sticker on the mirror that specifies it is "Imported Petit Points by Evans." The puff also has the name Evans. With no other mark, the collector can rest assured this one was made by Evans.

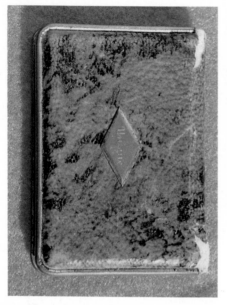

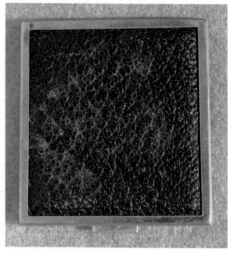

Small, square compact with leather insert in top. $25-$30.

Imitation leather, worn on corners, contains beveled mirror, powder, and rouge compartments. $25-$35.

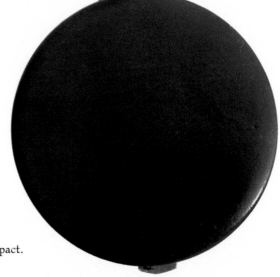

Black Lin Bren vinyl-covered compact. $30-$45.

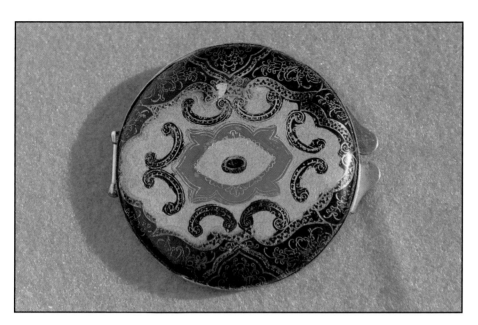

Leather covered compact, colorful design, unmarked. $45-$60.

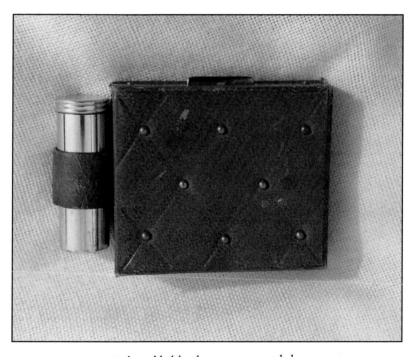

Nail studded leather compact with lipstick on side. Only mark is Genuine Leather. $75-$90.

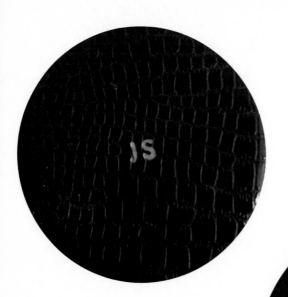

Leather compact, monogrammed J S. $45-$55.

Navy leather compact, monogrammed ESS, No mark except USA and a patent number. $40-$50.

Red leather Lin Bren compact, Mary on back. $30-$45.

Pink fabric Lin Bren compact. $30-$40.

Brown leather, Evans compact. $40-$55.

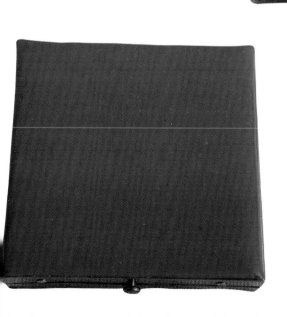

Square red leather Dorset compact. $40-$60.

83

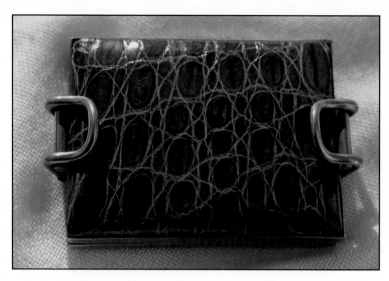

Alligator compact made in Argentina. $75-$100.

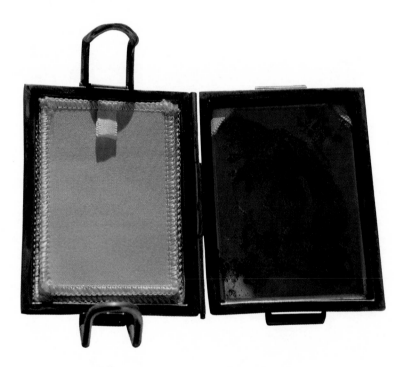

Alligator compact opens from the sides.

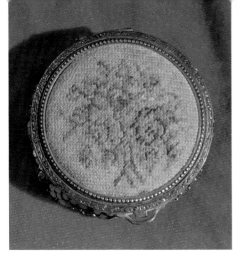

Petit point insert in top. Evans. $55-$75.

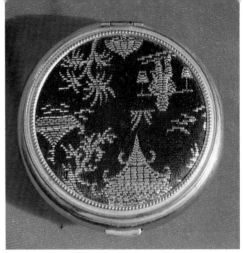

Lin Bren compact with embroidered insert in top. $50-$65.

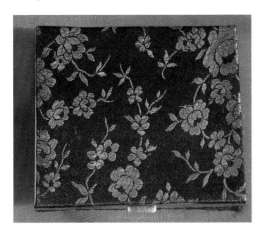

Brocade covered compact, silver design on black, unmarked. $50-$65.

Petit point insert, unmarked. $50-$65.

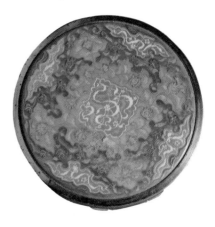

Coty powder compact. $35-$45.

Imitation tortoise shell compact with petit point top made in France. $65-$75.

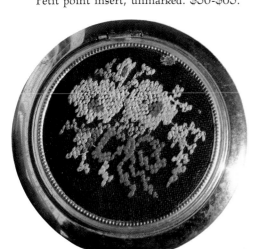

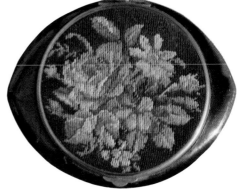

Chapter Nine:
Military Insignias

During the early part of the forties thousands of young men were uprooted from their homes and sent to military camps and bases all around the country to be trained for World War II. This meant they were hundreds, maybe thousands, of miles from their families and their girlfriends. No matter how far away they were, they still remembered the ruling of the mothers—only candy, perfume, flowers, and compacts were appropriate gifts to give a girl. Since flowers were almost entirely out of the question, that only left three choices. Perfume was easy enough to ship, but candy could melt, if sent to a southern climate by slow mail. So, there was nothing safe and reasonably priced left to send but compacts, and they were easy to acquire and easy to send. The Post Exchanges on every base had a plentiful supply of compacts, most with the insignias of the men serving there. The compacts were usually in a box which made it easy to wrap and send. Prices, especially in the PX, were very reasonable so the young men could send their girls as many compacts as they wanted. The girls were happy to be remembered so often. But perhaps the most important thing was the fact that so many of the military compacts had compartments behind the mirror so he could send a new picture of himself at regular intervals.

They might have had military insignias, but like all compacts, the bodies were made of various materials. Some were goldtone, others enameled, while an Evans has been found made of leather. One military type compact has been seen which appears to be made of some kind of hard plastic, and was made in the shape of the dress caps worn by the servicemen at that time. So many military compacts were made and sold during the war that they are still reasonably plentiful, but like everything else in antiquedom they are widely scattered. It is possible to find several in a show or mall, yet visit a dozen others without seeing one.

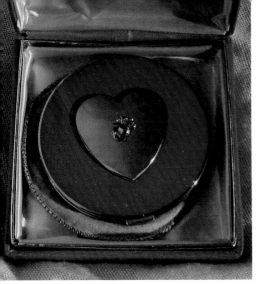

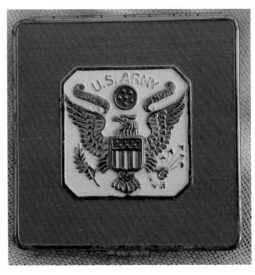

Beautiful red enameled top with goldtone heart topped with a Marine insignia. Still in box from New York jeweler. Never been used. Compact and puff marked Darling, which is believed to be the trademark. $125-$150.

Red background with framed white U. S. Army insignia. World War II vintage. Maker unknown. $35-$50.

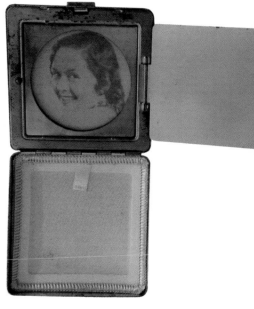

Black enamel top and bottom on copper case. Due to shortage of materials during wartime copper was used instead of goldtone or other materials. Military insignia in left corner. American Maid trademark. $20-$25.

Inside of compact (above) showing how mirror swings out to reveal picture compartment.

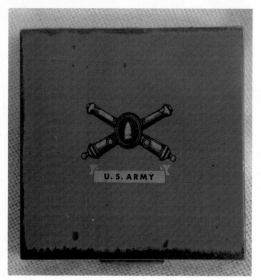 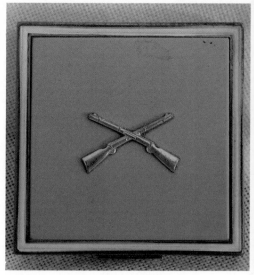

Inexpensive compact with U. S. Army
Artillery insignia. World War II. $15-
$20.

Better quality compact, Infantry insignia on blue enameled background.
Never used. Evans trademark. $25-
$35.

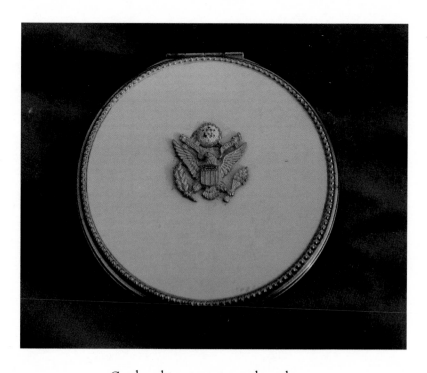

Good quality compact, powder only.
Never used. Military insignia. $35-$45.

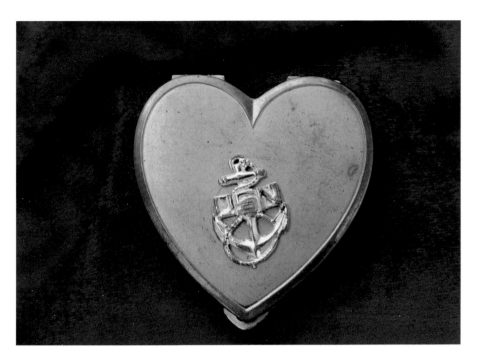

Heart-shaped compacts are not too plentiful. This one has Navy insignia. Unmarked. $45-$65.

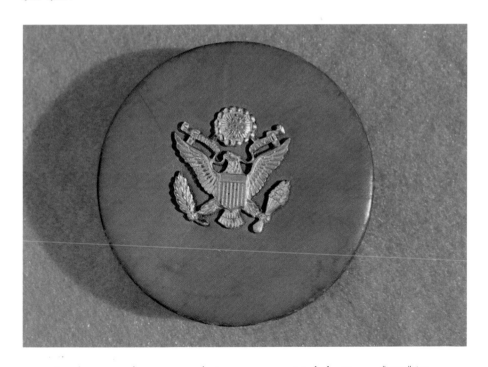

Leather covered compact with Army insignia. Made by Evans. $45-$65.

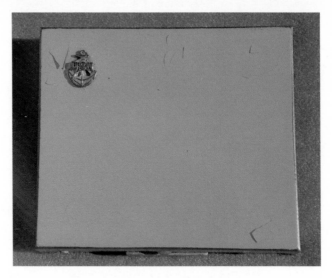

Blue enamel top and bottom on copper
ground. Navy insignia in left corner.
Picture frame behind mirror. World War
II vintage. Unmarked. $20-$25.

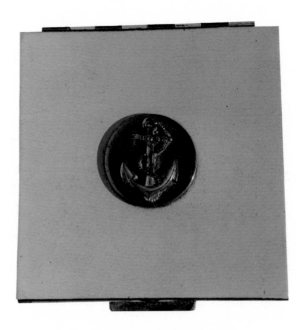

Square, white compact with Navy insignia. Rex Fifth Avenue trademark. $30-
$40.

Chapter Ten:
Miscellaneous

Miscellaneous is still the most magnificient word we know to pull together all the odds and ends of any subject. In the case of compacts it is even more useful as there are lots of different sizes, shapes, designs, and materials. Examples include one with a wooden case or body, one made out of aluminum, several with Eastern Star insignias, and one with a Shrine emblem. There are fan shapes, heart shapes, and one in the shape of a basket complete with handle. And there is one with a cameo on top that doesn't quite fit into the jeweled top category, although it does have a design on top. The word miscellaneous forms an umbrella to covers all the various styles.

The compact made of aluminum is a real challenge. It is the only one we have seen made of that material, but if one style was made, chances are others were as well, although it's doubtful enough could be found to give aluminum compacts their own category. It is bright enough to pass for silver, but it isn't. What appears to be a helmeted Roman soldier is on the front with a circle of stars around the edge, and the back has a well designed eagle in a circle with a wreath and stars around the outside on it. It is not marked in any way, nor was there a puff found that might have helped to identify it. It is not all that unusual when all the different kinds of compacts are taken into consideration, it is just one of the dozens that seem to defy a single classification.

Then there is the Art Deco design, a compact with yellow, orange, silver and black stripes and half stripes. Enough heart-shaped examples could probably be found if one looked long enough, but they are so varied that most of them will fit into other categories. The one included here has a blue enameled top with a smaller goldtone heart in the top left hand corner. The balance is a nice goldtone. No name could be found on either the puff or the compact itself.

Another item that has been included is not a compact at all, it was simply found with a collection of compacts. It is a small purse 2 by 3.5 inches, made of bone and what appears to be silver trim. The body or foundation is brass. When opened there are four compartments, each lined with red silk. The ends that open out appear to be made of leather. A small clasp on the center marked *Paris* closes off two compartments, leaving two. The name on the front is illegible. This is just one of the many "necessary things" women carried in their purses half a century ago.

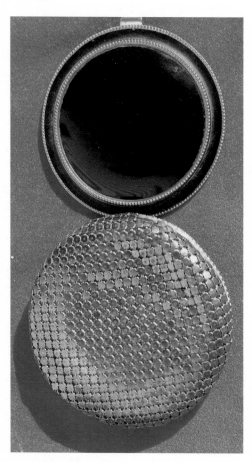

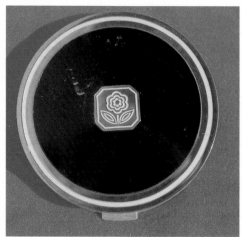

Jean La Solle compact. $40-$55.

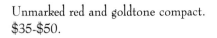

Black enameled top, mesh bottom. Unmarked. $50-$65.

Unmarked red and goldtone compact. $35-$50.

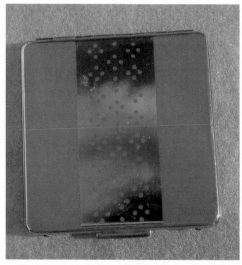

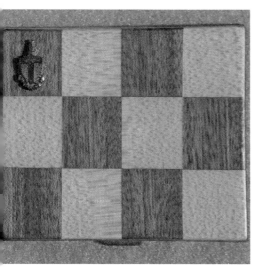

Unmarked compact with wooden top. $40-$50.

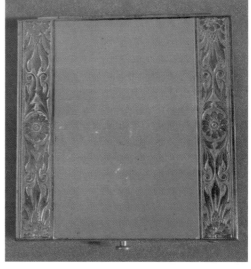

Goldtone panels down the side, light blue center. $40-$50.

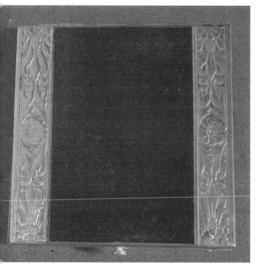

Same style with dark blue center. $40-$50.

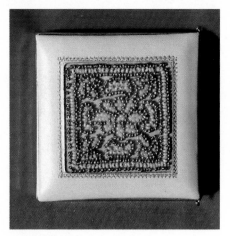

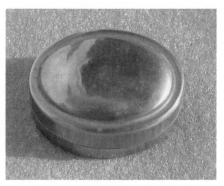

Beaded leather compact by Daniel. $65-$75.

Small brass container, originally had cream rouge. $10-$12.

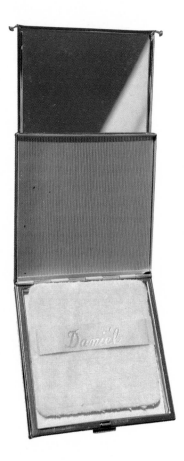

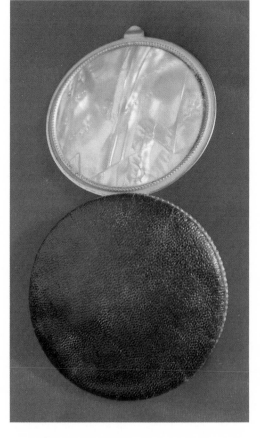

Mirror pulls out of top.

Celluloid top, leather bottom, unmarked. $35-$45.

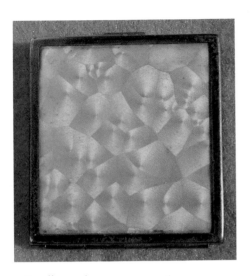 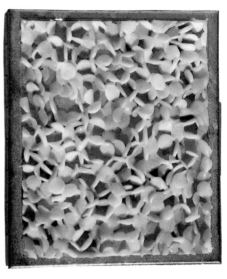

Small, powder compact, pink insert in cover. $25-$35.

Unmarked compact with multi-colored top. $30-$40.

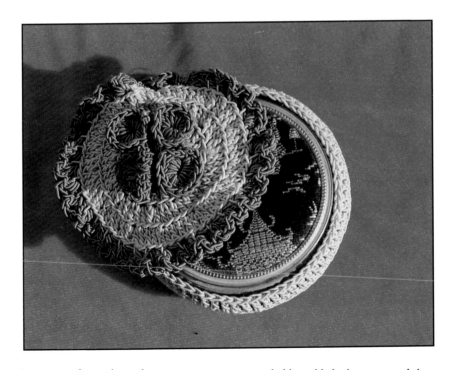

Directions for making this compact case was probably published in some of the needlework magazines. Case only $10-$15.

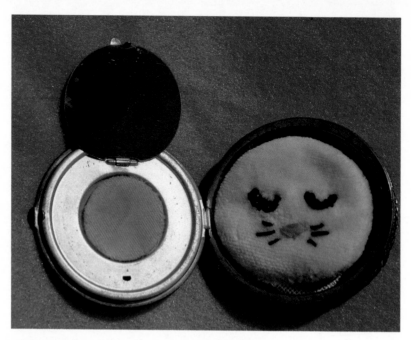

Embroidered cat's faces on compact puffs were also popular. Puff only $8-$12.

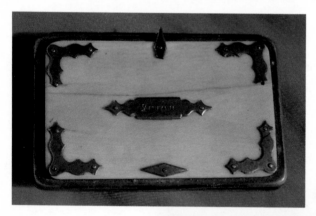

Small, bone-covered purse decorated with silver found in compact drawer. $45-$55.

Houbigant powder, rouge, and lipstick compact. $75-$85.

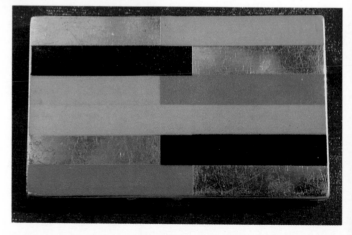

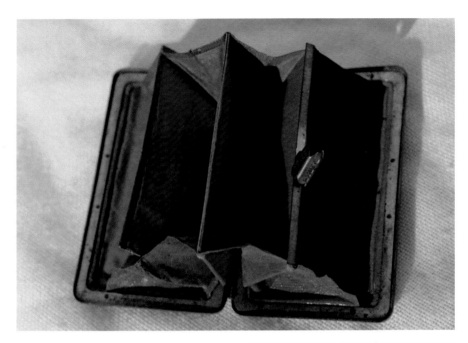

Four silk and leather sections inside
bone purse, Paris on inside fastener.

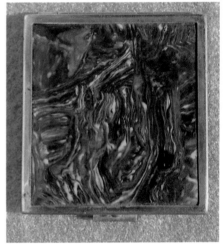

Small compact with plastic insert in
top. $25-$30.

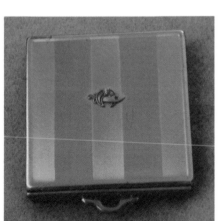

No mark except patent number. Shrine
emblem on top. $50-$75.

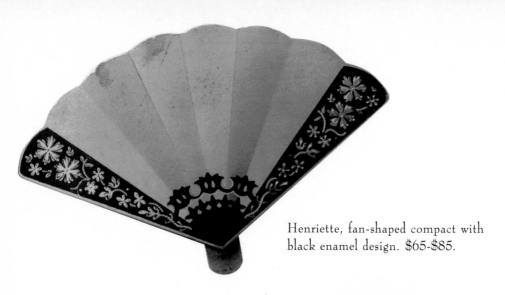

Henriette, fan-shaped compact with black enamel design. $65-$85.

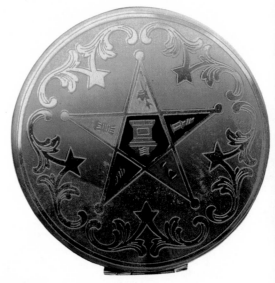

Elgin American, round compact with Eastern Star insignia. $70-$85.

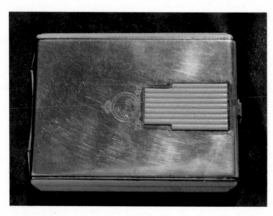

Goldtone top on sky blue compact. $35-$45.

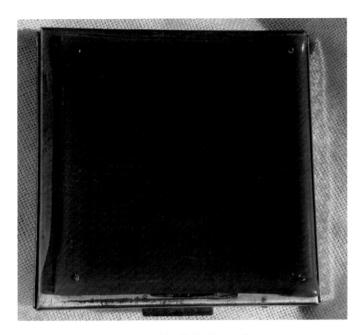

Rex goldtone with celluloid top. $40-$50.

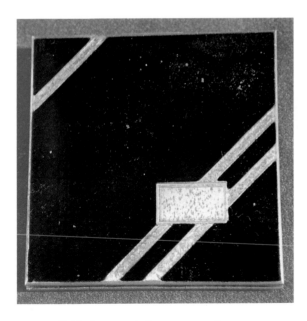

Zell black enameled compact with goldtone decorations. Instructions inside for using Sift-Proof Zell. $45-$65.

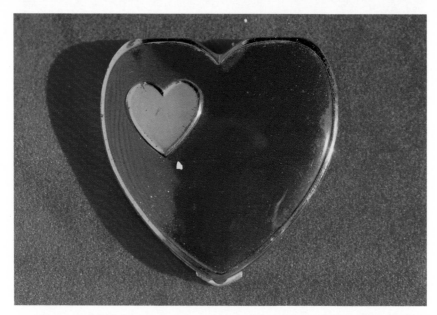

Blue enameled heart-shaped compact with goldtone heart. $50-$65.

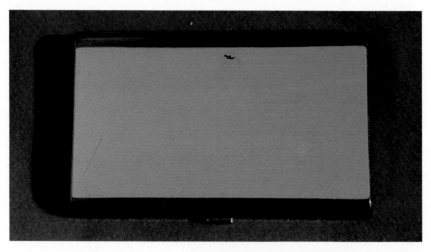

Oblong enameled powder and rouge compact. $40-$60.

Oblong, black enameled compact with rhinestone design. $30-$45.

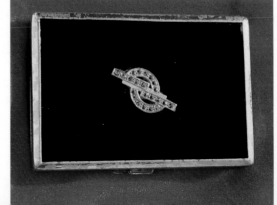

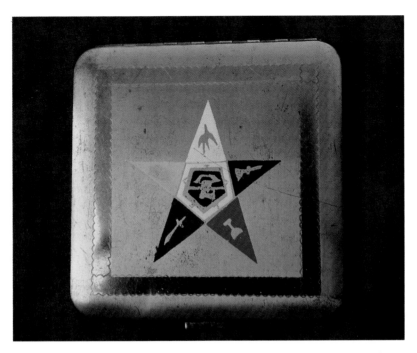

Dorset marked compact, Dorset Rex puff, Eastern Star insignia. $75-$90.

White enamel compact. $25-$35.

Chapter Eleven:
Mother-of-Pearl Compacts

For a century or more mother-of-pearl was a favorite form of decoration, especially for toilet articles, the handles of knives and forks, and small pieces of jewelry. That is due, it is believed, to its beautiful iridescence which resembles pearls. And well it should, as mother-of-pearl was obtained from the shells of several types of mussels including the pearl oyster. Using the shells of the ones that were suitable, the inside was removed and cut into thin sheets ideal for decorating various items. The pieces which would be used on knives, forks, and manicure tools were left solid. Today, the majority of mussel shells come from Japan and surrounding areas, as they are the biggest producers of fresh water pearls, but this was not always the case. In the early days mussel shells were obtained from many areas, any area with warm waters including the Mediterranean Sea, where some of the most choice ones were obtained.

For about fifty years, from around 1880 to about 1930, the favorite pieces of jewelry, for those who could afford it, were pearls, genuine cultured pearls. The choice was strands of pearls to be worn around the neck. It could be anything from one to a half dozen strands, but the favorites were three to five strands. It is next to impossible today to find a picture of a well-to-do matron or dowager who does not have on a pearl necklace. Young girls wore one strand, and always in their wedding pictures. Since pearls were associated with the affluent and the socially correct, it is only natural that the mother-of-pearl compacts and carryalls became so popular. Judging by the ads they were a little more expensive than the run-of-the-mill compacts, but still affordable for the average person. Apparently the presumption that only the rich can wear pearls still exists in some quarters, if we are to judge by the price seen on run-of-the-mill, mother-of-pearl compacts seen in an antique mall recently. Most will be priced in the $25 to $35 range, in our area, but this particular one, a very plain one, was priced $200, while another seen recently was priced over $200.

Whether it was an effort to make compacts that would be less expensive (during the Depression), or simply the fact that genuine mother-of-pearl was less plentiful and more expensive is unknown. But it is known that during the thirties an imitation mother-of-pearl was being made. It was described as being as iridescent as the real thing, but less expensive. It is usually easy to distinguish the real from the imitation primarily because most of the imitation pieces are solid, that is the top of the compact is in one piece.

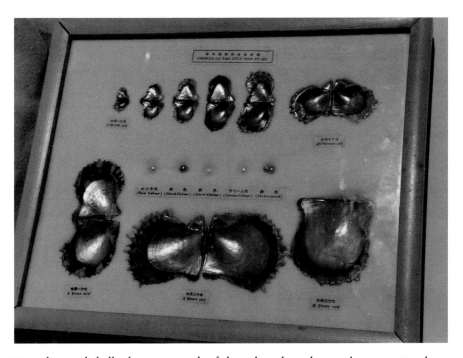

Framed mussel shells showing growth of the cultured pearl over the years. Pearls were found inside some while certain types could be used to make mother-of-pearl.

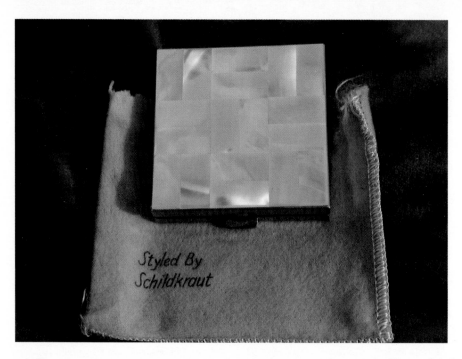

Small mother-of-pearl compact with "Genuine Mother-of-Pearl by Schildkraut" label on mirror. Unused. $45-$70.

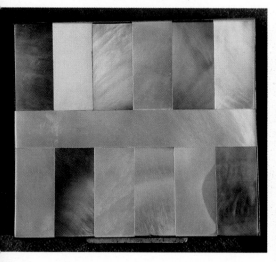

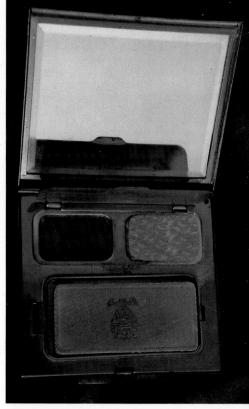

Mother-of-pearl compact by Foster. Beveled mirror. $95-$135.

Inside of Foster compact showing compartments for powder, rouge, and cream lipstick.

104

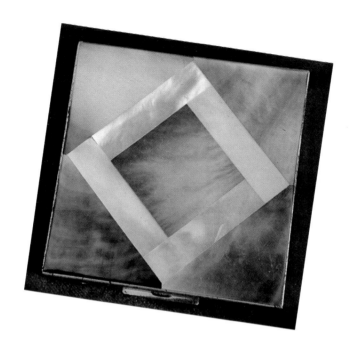

Light and dark pieces of mother-of-pearl were used. Only mark is Z (could be Zell) and U.S.A. $60-$85.

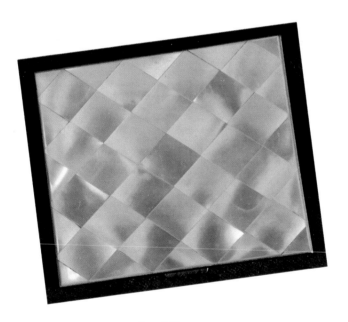

Compact with a different arrangement of the mother-of-pearl. Unmarked. $55-$90.

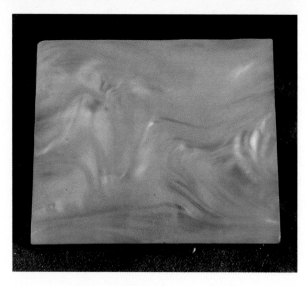

Imitation mother-of-pearl compact, unmarked. $25-$35.

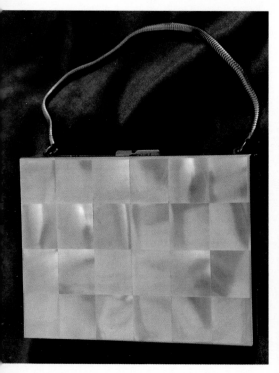

Open showing arrangement of powder,
lipstick, and comb.

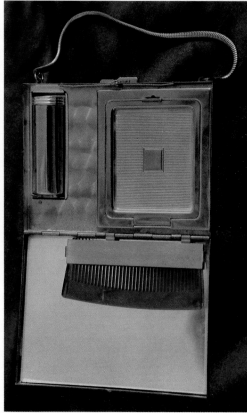

Almost square mother-of-pearl carryall,
double opening, back is cigarette case,
snake chain handle. Unmarked. $115-
$150.

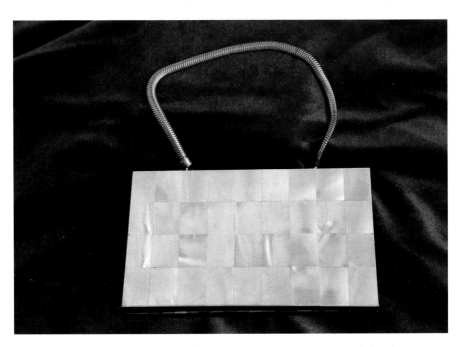

Carryall, one side mother-of-pearl, single opening, cigarette case behind mirror. "Marhill Genuine Mother-of-Pearl" label on mirror. $150-$200.

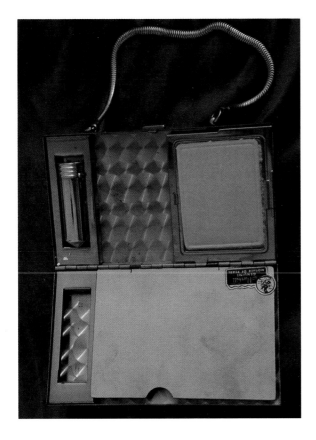

Inside showing label.

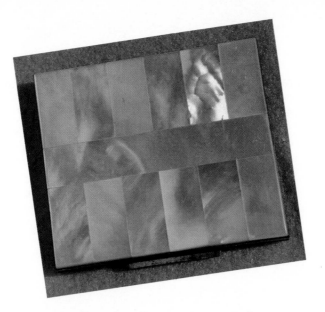

Mother-of-pearl compact, unmarked.
$45-$70.

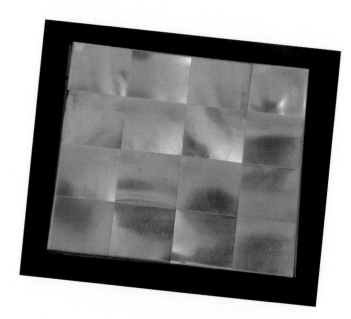

Compact with label "Sam Fink Genuine Mother-of-Pearl." $55-$85.

Chapter Twelve:
Novelties

For lack of a more descriptive word to cover all the different types of compacts used in this category, we settled on novelties. Actually there aren't that many novel ones here, but the majority of them are more unusual and more interesting than those used in the old catch-all miscellaneous category.

One of these compacts that absolutely defies classification is a thin goldtone example without a mark of any kind except "Louis C. Tiffany - favrile" etched across the top. It came out of the estate of an average Maine family. All of the family members who might have known anything about it were deceased when the estate was sold, so there was nobody left to ask about it. After several years of study and questioning dealers and collectors alike, the answer seems to lie in one of three possibilities. It is possible Tiffany had a few of these compacts made to give to special favrile customers, or it is possible—but not very probable— that some compact maker added the information in an effort to sell more compacts. But there would probably have been a lawsuit unless the manufacturer had the blessings of Tiffany. The only other answer we came up with was that some husband either etched the words or had them etched to produced a very special gift for his wife who collected Tiffany favrile.

For sometime before and after the turn of the present century women wore watches, not the popular wrist watch of the twenties and thereafter, but small closed case watches that could be worn either on a chain around their necks, or pinned on their jacket lapels. These watches were very popular and the majority of women owned one, which explains why so many compacts were made later in the shape of those early watches. Incidentally, the compacts could also be worn like the earlier watches. In fact, Lilly Daché made one around the thirties or forties that only had the numerals around the outside like a watch, but the inside was used for perfume rather than powder and paint. One of the most unusual of the watch-shaped compacts has a amber colored disk in the front with people in it. There is no indication of the maker except the puff with the Max Factor logo. Since neither the pressed powder nor the puff has been used, it is reasonably safe to assume the puff is the original. Another that could easily pass for a watch is almost identical in both shape and design to the majority of old watches. There is no mark, nor is there a puff. Several were made with small watches about the size and shape of the later wrist watch in the top with the watch facing out. One Evans is shaped like a modified camel-back trunk completed with metal straps. The mirror folds up to allow the watch to be wound.

Another novel idea was the musical compact. One example included here is an Elgin American that plays the tune *Let Me Call You Sweetheart*. During the romantic period in which this was made, compacts like this one would have been an all time favorite.

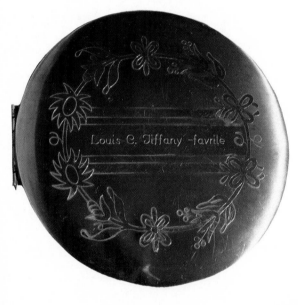

Unmarked except for the Louis C. Tiffany - Favile. Could be a gift, advertising, or perhaps some engraver did it for a special collecting friend. $100-$150.

Attractive Max Factor watch-shaped compact, opens with stem. $95-$125.

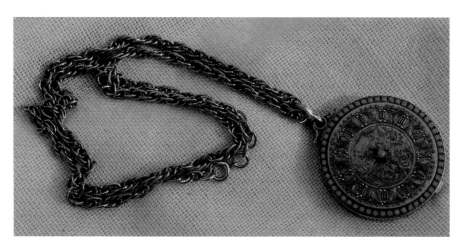

Perfume has always been very important to the ladies. Lilly Daché designed this watch-shaped necklace as a perfume holder. $100-$150

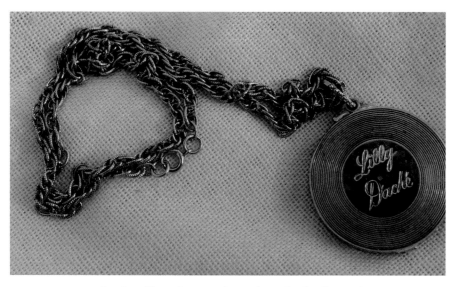

Back of necklace showing the trademark of Lilly Daché.

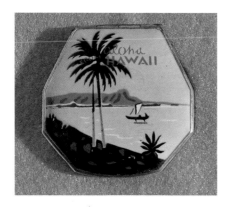

Inexpensive souvenir compact from Hawaii. $15-$20.

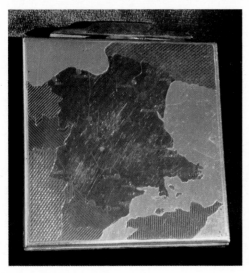

Compact with map of France, Made in France. $55-$75.

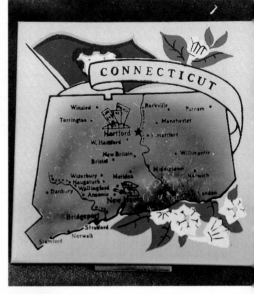

Elgin American souvenir compact from Connecticut, Myrtle engraved on back. $50-$60.

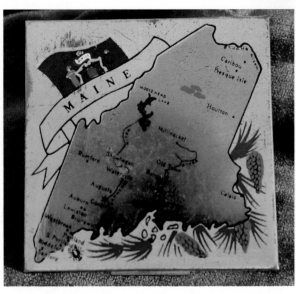

Elgin American compact, Maine souvenir. $50-$60.

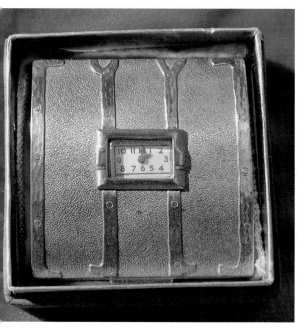

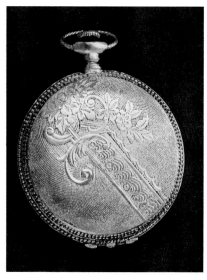

Evans compact, strapped like a trunk, watch in top, still in Evans gift box. $125-$150.

More realistic looking watch compact, unmarked but similar to Max Factor. $60-$75.

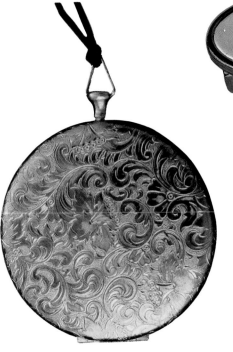

Perfume bottle in fancy case, Germaine Monteil perfume. $40-$50.

Watch-shaped compact. $50-$75.

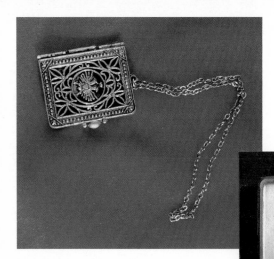

Bracelets like this were also used for perfume. $25-$30.

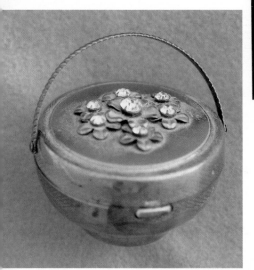

Illinois Watch Case Company compact with powder, rouge, and a watch that still runs. $150-$185.

Compact shaped like a basket. $50-$65.

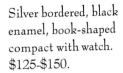

Silver bordered, black enamel, book-shaped compact with watch. $125-$150.

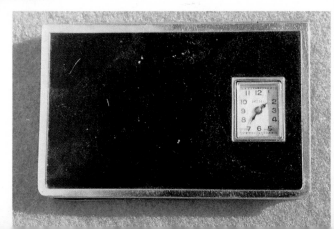

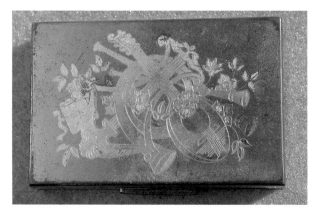

Elgin American musical compact.
$200-$235.

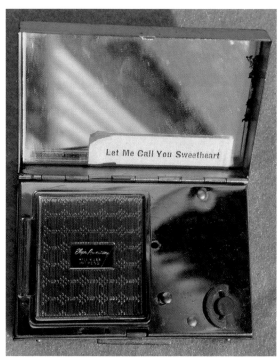

Still plays *Let Me Call You Sweetheart*.

Henriette fan-shaped compact, black
enamel top, goldtone bottom. $65-$85.

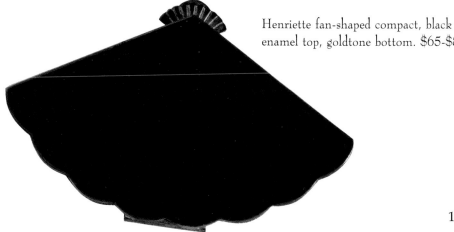

Collecting and displaying compacts is the fun part; trying to categorize them can sometimes be difficult as one of the problems in that field is the fact you may not have but one or two that seems to fit each category. Then you decide on a category titled Pictorials that according to the dictionary means "pertaining to, characterized by, or composed of pictures,"—and you can use nearly anything in it.

Volupté made a wide variety of compacts, carryalls, and cigarette cases with the same design—lions attacking antelopes, elephants, and a variety of birds that could fit into this category. The cases appear to be made of brass rather than lightweight goldtone, and there is quite a bit of color applied. So many of these were made that everybody must have seen at least one. But one of those shown in this category is not as unusual for the different arrangement inside as it is for the old price tags stuck on the mirror. It appears to have been written or printed with an ink pen. It gives the date, Nov. 18, 1954; describes the object as a portmanteau, the old name for leather luggage, although the same name has been found in catalogs to identify some types of leather purses; and the price which is $25. The inside of this one is different than most of the other carryalls as it only has a place for powder with the space above it divided into two compartments, one for pressed rouge, the other for lipstick. That takes up half of one side while the other side is empty. It doesn't even have a cover. This space could possibly have been designed for money. The other side, behind the mirror is also empty, but it was probably meant to be used as a cigarette case.

Another compact that defies classification, not because of the portrait on the front but because of its strange style, is the small blue enamel one with two mirrors, one on the inside and another covering the entire back. There must have been another section that fit on the back although several similar compacts have been seen and they all have a mirror that covers the entire back. It is questionable what purpose another section would have filled as there is already a place for both powder and rouge in the top.

Not too many zipper closure compacts have been seen although the one illustrated here has a label in the bottom that declares "This is one of a series of twelve delightful originals by Warner of Hollywood." The odd-shaped puff that has never been used and is certainly the original has the name Lady Vanity. That would more than likely be the name under which Warner marketed the compacts. Another unusual feature of this zippered compact is the fact the name Annette Honeywell, the artist, is printed on the front underneath the dancer. She was probably a well-known stage or studio dancer. Several other types of compacts were made depicting dancers.

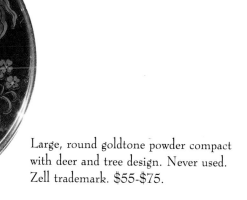

Square goldtone compact with enameled dancing couple. Unmarked. $40-$60.

Large, round goldtone powder compact with deer and tree design. Never used. Zell trademark. $55-$75.

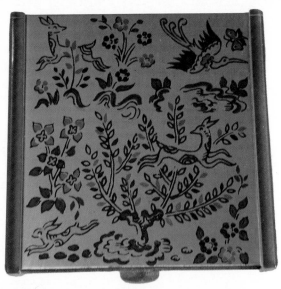

Large, square powder compact, animal design, unmarked. $50-$65.

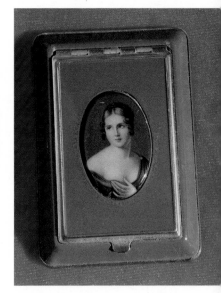

Blue enamel with portrait of Victorian lady. Powder and rouge wells, mirror under lid and on back. Unmarked. $40-$50.

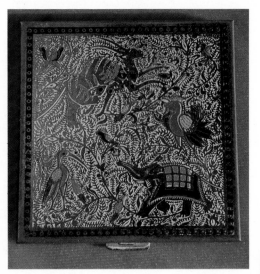

Volupté used this design on powder only compacts, carryalls, and cigarette cases. $45-$60.

Blue enameled compact with birds and flower design. Unmarked. $35-$45.

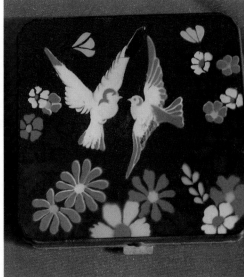

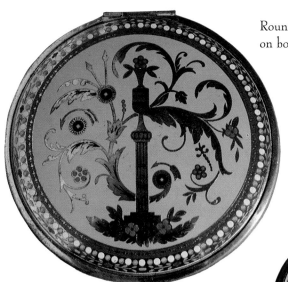

Round Volupté compact, same design on both sides. $45-$65.

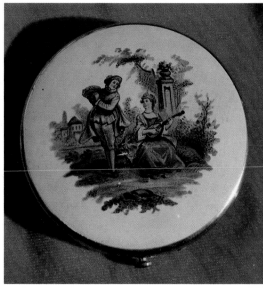

Small, round compact with silver dancing figures on green ground, sift thru powder compartment, Terri trademark. $25-$35.

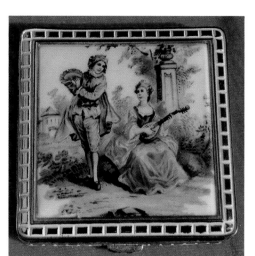

Rex Fifth Avenue powder only compact. Never used. $50-$65.

Rex used the same design on this less expensive compact. $35-$45.

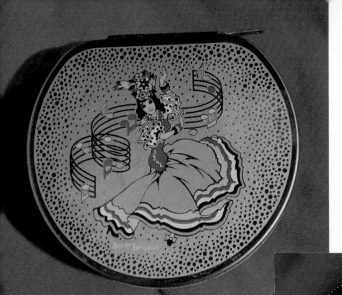

Zipper closure compact, one of a set of twelve made by Warner of Hollywood under the trade name Lady Vanity. One of the very few compacts with the artist's name. In this case Annette Honeywell. $90-$115.

Showing inside of compact.

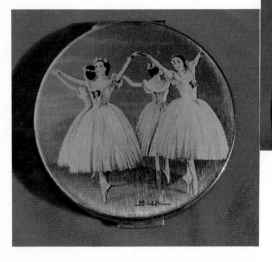

Stratton dancing girls compact, artist signed. $65-$75.

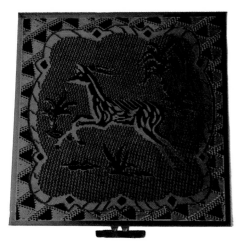

Volupté used animal designs on many of their compacts. $50-$75.

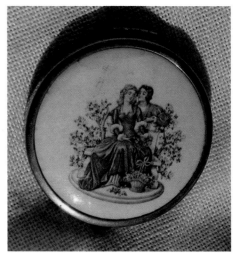

Small, Yardley, powder only compact. $20-$25.

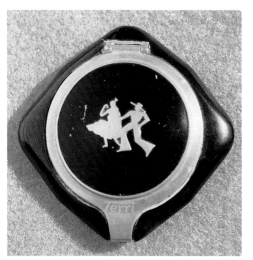

Small Terri compact with dancing figures. $15-$20.

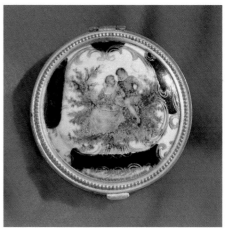

Small powder only compact. $25-$30.

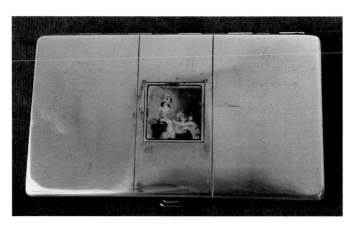

Yardley compact, has name on the back, between powder and paint compartments, and in powder well. $25-$30.

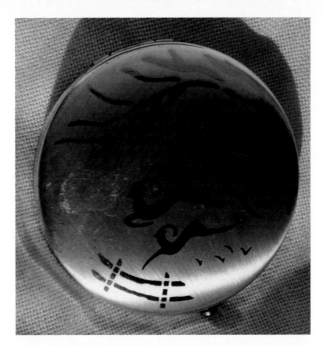

Compact decorated with goldtone gazelles, Dorset trademark. $25-$35.

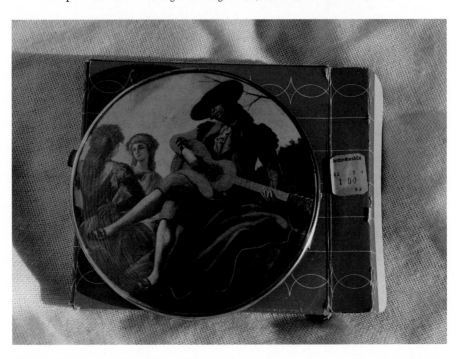

The most interesting thing about this compact is the price tag on the original box. There is no date but it appears to be around 1950. At that time this Zell compact was priced $1 by Jordon Marsh Company. $50-$65.

Chapter Fourteen:
Powder Boxes, Musical and Plain

The demand for face powder, both pressed and loose, really began in earnest in the twenties, and by the forties was big business. Talking movies had begun in 1926. This was a whole new form of entertainment because prior to this time about the only thing the young people had was either the phonograph or the radio, which meant they had to stay in their own parlors. Movies opened up a whole new world for them, where they felt free—free of the watchful eyes of mothers who set stern rules for their daughters when they entertained their boyfriends at home. According to some of the women who were young girls at the time, they might leave home with little or no makeup and return the same way, but once they got to the powder room at the theatre, they applied as much makeup as they wanted, usually as much as the actress on the screen seemed to be wearing. It wasn't as professionally done as that on the actress, but it made them feel they were equally as glamorous, they said.

The use of makeup was new to them, at least the type and style they saw on their favorite movie stars. Apparently, it was important to lots of people because looking through magazines from that era it is noticeable how many makeup people from the movie studios and from the modeling agencies were interviewed or wrote articles about the secrets of applying makeup correctly. The modeling agencies were important because so many stars found their way into the movies by the modeling route.

Generally the ladies used their loose face powder from two different containers. They could use it directly from the box that was usually kept on their vanity, and by filling their compacts. Or they could buy fancy powder and puff boxes that were made in a variety of styles and materials. That was an era of dresser sets that might be simple with only a hand mirror, comb, brush, hair receiver, and powder box, or they might include a half dozen more pieces. One set seen recently had a pair of matching candleholders. The sets could be made of any material, but celluloid, especially the white celluloid sets which were often marked French Ivory, seemed to be among the favorites. This opinion is based on the fact so many can be found today.

Then there were the musical powder and puff boxes. The majority of those seen today are made of metal. For instance, nine musical powder and puff boxes were shown in the 1932 Wallenstein Mayer catalog. They were a wholesale jewelry company located in Cincinnati. Prices ranged from $7.50 to $14 each (wholesale), or about the same price seen on them now in the malls in our area. They are much higher in other areas. In the catalog they were described as "Combination powder and puff box, fancy brocade finish metal with hand painted porcelain in cover. Automatically plays an up-to-date air." This one with painted porcelain in the cover is very similar to those shown in the illustrations. It was priced $8 wholesale in 1932.

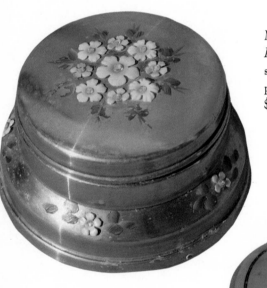

Musical powder box plays *Brahms Lullaby* when lid is raised, large box, small container in top for powder and/or puff. Applied flowers on metal box. $25-$35.

Celluloid powder box from dresser set. Marked Pyralin, Arlington. $5-$9.

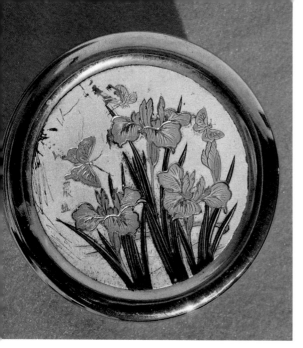

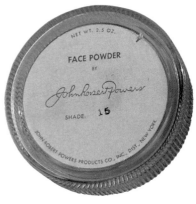

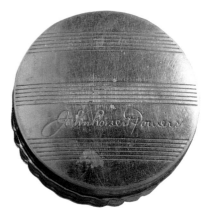

Late porcelain powder jar. Lid decorated with Chokin, an ancient art used on Samurai armor years ago. Made in Japan. Artist initials under largest butterfly. $25-$35.

Movie make-up artists, talent agencies, or anyone closely associated with the business of making women beautiful might produce or have made all types of cosmetics. These empty John Robert Powers face powder jars were probably saved because they could be used again and again. $10-$18.

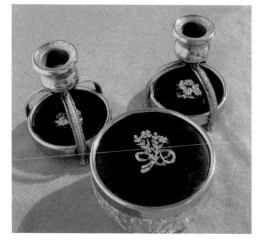

Glass powder jar with marcasite-type decoration on black top. Jar and candlesticks were part of a dresser set, but candlesticks were unusual in those sets. Maker unknown. Powder jar $20-$25, The three pieces $40-$60.

125

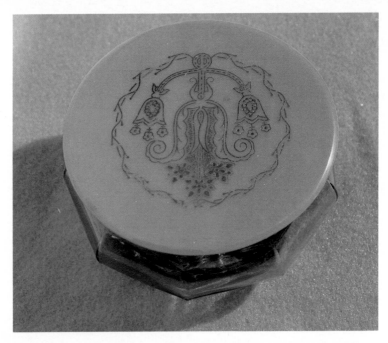

Amber glass powder jar, celluloid top. Part of dresser set. $7-$9.

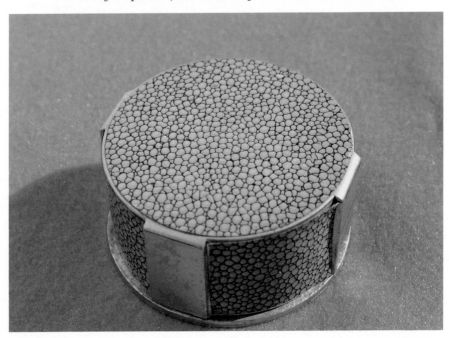

Unopened box of Gemey face powder, made by Richard Hudnut, circa 1950. Loose powder like this could be put into compacts, used from the box, or put in powder jars. $9-$11.

Attractive powder box with Victorian-type girl on top. Originally filled with Ciara dusting powder made by Charles Revson, New York. When empty it could be used for face powder and puff. $6-$8.

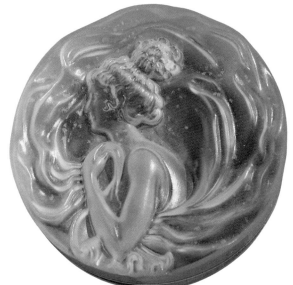

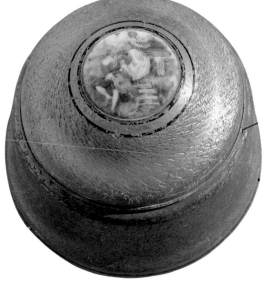

Unopened box of Deltah face powder. Handwritten on the top of the paper cover is the following: "You will appreciate the fragrant, velvety, clinging qualities of this pure silk-sifted face powder—another fascinating creation by Deltah." Metal box with hinged lid. $15-$25.

In 1932 The Wallenstein Mayer Company, Cincinnati, Ohio wholesaler jewelry firm, offered a page of this type combination powder and puff boxes. Prices varied from $7.50 to $9 each wholesale. They were described as "Fancy brocade finish metal with hand painted porcelain in cover." They automatically played one "up-to-date air," according to the advertisement. They played the tune automatically after someone had wound them up. Four inches in diameter at bottom, 3.25 inches tall. $35-$50.

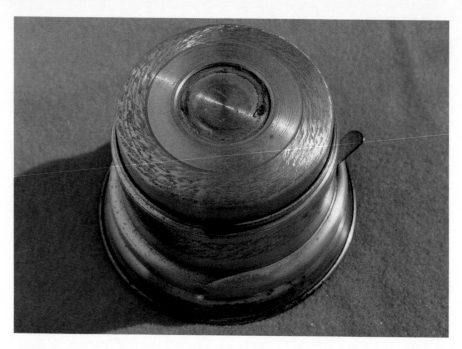

Same type musical powder and puff box. Hand painted porcelain missing from cover. $20-$25.

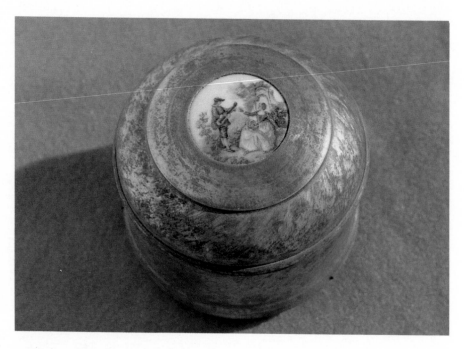

Same type Wallenstein Mayer musical powder and puff box, but larger. 5.5 inch bottom diameter, 4 inches tall. $35-$55.

Chapter Fifteen:
Purses, Fitted or Matching

Items in this category can run the gamut from fine brocade purses in varying sizes to alligator envelope bags and portmanteaus. The portmanteau, mentioned earlier, was advertised in catalogs around the turn of the century. It was described as perfect for women to take shopping or for travel. The so-called envelope-type purse, both leather and fabric, became famous in the thirties and forties. If any one person helped to make it so popular, it would be Joan Crawford, one of the movie queens of that period. She seemed to always wear a tailored suit and carry an envelope-type purse. The alligator items aren't the most popular now due to the fact many people dislike the killing of any reptile or fur bearing animal to make clothing and accessories. Maybe we shouldn't kill anymore, but there is no reason to destroy the things we already have, we can at least save them. For this reason the prices of any reptile accessory will vary, sometimes greatly, from one area to another.

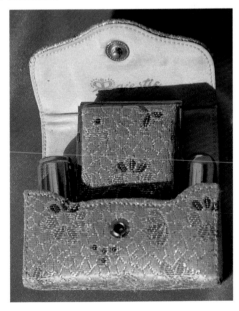

Small, fitted brocade purse by Majestic, matching cover on compact, comb, two lipsticks. $100-$125.

Another fitted purse (or is it a carryall?) is the imitation leather, zippered example. It is really too large to fit into the average purse, yet is not pretty enough to be carried alone. It would be perfect for some chores as it has all the necessary items like comb, mirror, nail file, coins, and compact, and it would fit perfectly in a large coat pocket. Generally, the name on the compact is the name of the manufacturer, but in this case it is almost certain the original compact was removed and replaced with this more expensive Richard Hudnut.

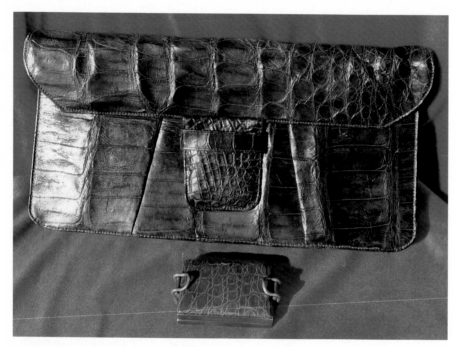

Circa 1940 alligator purse and compact made in Argentina. Purse $95-$125, compact $75-$100.

White top grain cowhide billfold and matching compact. Beaded design on top. Daniel trademark. Pair $95-$135.

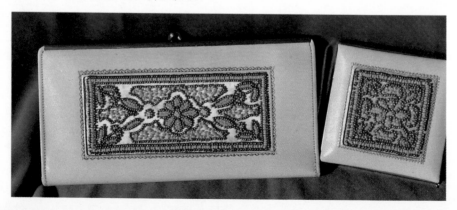

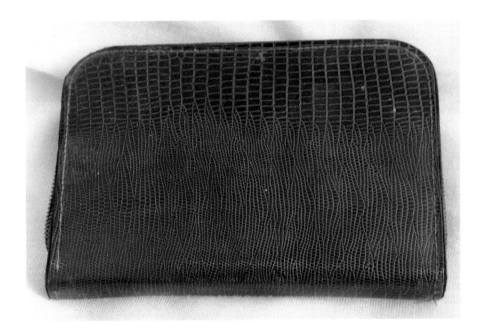

Leather fitted purse or case with zipper all around. $95-$100.

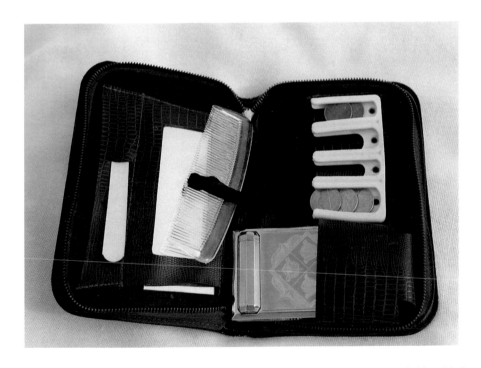

Inside of fitted purse. Has rather expensive Richard Hudnut compact, probably added later.

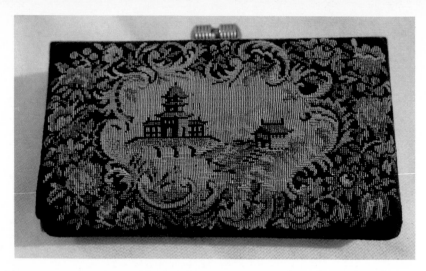

Tapestry purse or case, 3.5 by 6 inches. Has compact, lipstick, comb, and mirror. $75-$85.

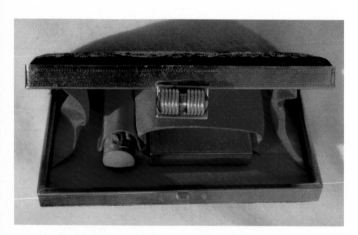

Inside showing contents.

Satin brocade clutch or case. Only identification is the name Quinlan on compact. $100-$150.

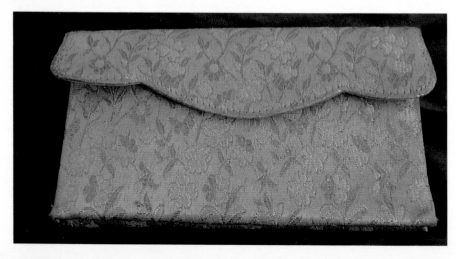

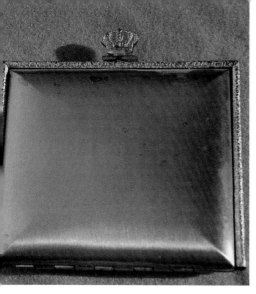

Goldtone clutch or evening bag. Only
had Foster compact when found. $75-
$100.

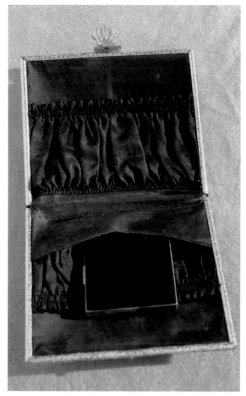

Inside showing compartments.

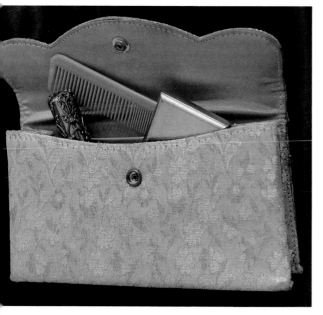

Inside of clutch or case. Lipstick and maybe the compact
was added later.

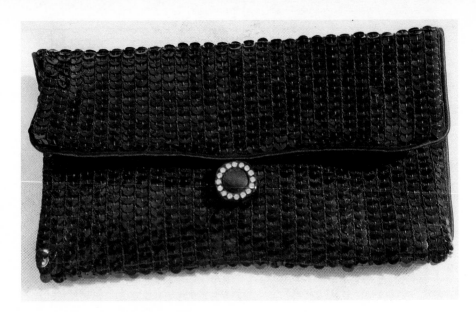

Norell black sequined evening bag.
$150-$175.

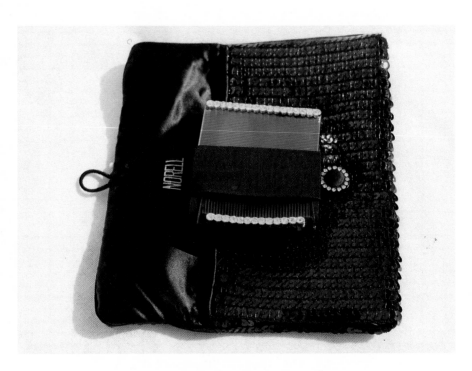

Bag fitted with rhinestone encrusted
compact and comb.

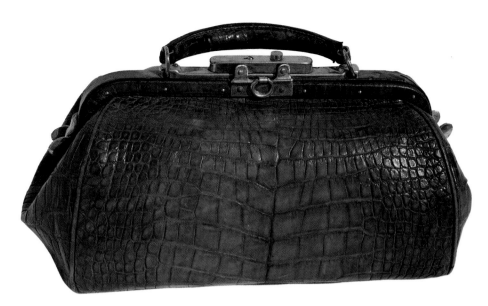

In the early part of this century this alligator portmanteau was advertised as perfect for shopping or for traveling. $200-$250.

Volupté goldtone carryall fitted with powder, lipstick, cigarette case, mirror, and compartment for money and keys. $100-$135.

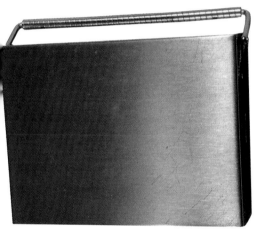

Tapestry clutch or bag fitted with coin holder and compact. $55-$75.

Small, fitted Faille bag, goldtone ends. $100-$125 due to replacements.

Fitted with Evans compact and Max Factor lipstick, one or both are definitely replacements. Comb is original.

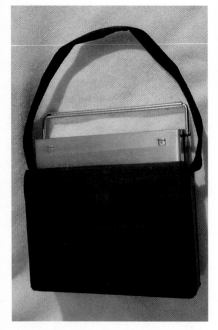

Volupté carryall that could be used alone or with the black faille case. Case has expandable pocket on back for money or keys. $125-$150.

Chapter Sixteen:
Silver Colored Compacts

Manufacturers have long known that they had to please the customer to stay in business, and if they didn't know previously, they soon learned that people have very strong ideas about what they like. Just like their choice in jewelry, there are people who prefer gold over silver or vise versa. Then there were women with the same preferences in the color of their compacts. For that reason the same style compact may be found in either silver or gold color. And to please those who couldn't make up their minds, they combined the two colors in some compacts.

This is even true in an Evans sterling compact, a basketweave design with the weavers in three colors, silver, gold, and bronze. Another interesting cross-over is the one advertised in 1949, maybe later, by Evans Case Company, North Attleboro, Massachusetts. It was described as the "bracelet-handled Coronation Carryall fitted with after-five indespensables." Some of these carryalls were made in goldtones while others were made in silver colored metals. In 1949 these carryalls were advertised for $36.50, a princely sum at that time. This was a time when most women were very fashion conscious; everything had to match. If they were wearing gold evening shoes, then the carryall had to be gold. Silver shoes demanded a silver carryall. This was a time when shoes and bags or carryall were the same color, there were no exceptions, unless the wearer didn't care about style.

The Elgin American compact with the birds on the cover is another strange use of colors. The silver outside is a combination of matte and glossy finish while the inside is goldtone. The small chain handled compact that is definitely 1920ish and made for the Flappers is not marked, but could possibly be sterling. Silver was quite inexpensive in those days, but not as inexpensive as some other materials. The cost factor could have played an important part in both the design and the color of most compacts. The two compacts with the work scenes, one farming and the other questionable, appears to be sterling and possibly is because as we have just said silver was not that expensive then. The one with the questionable scene is marked with only the word Denmark while the one with the Oriental farming scene is not marked at all. They are different in both style, shape, and workmanship so it is possible they were made in different areas. The original owner of the silver-colored Houbigant was so determined to take care of her compact, she made a lovely embroidered case to keep it in. Quite a few crocheted compact cases have been seen, but embroidered ones are scarce. The cases add to the value of the compact as the compact is usually in better condition, and then there is the lovely case it can be kept in for many more years.

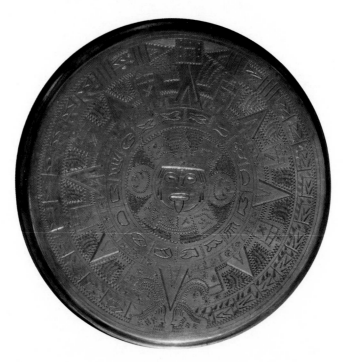

Sterling silver compact, Mexico. $150-$200.

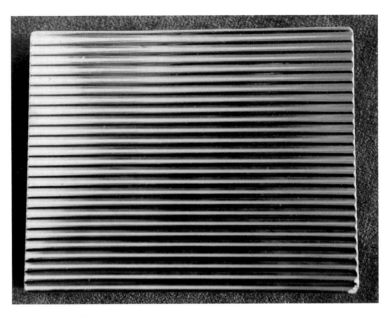

Silver colored compact, beveled mirror, fluffy puff, made in France. $50-$65.

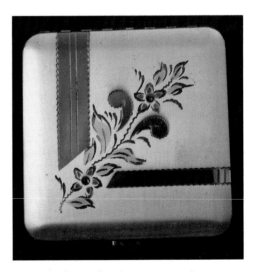

Dorset silver-colored compact with goldtone band and floral design. Still in gift box. $50-$70

Showing inside of compact.

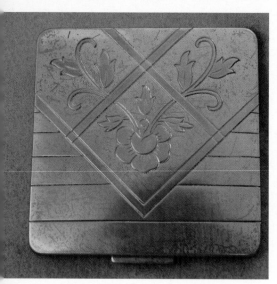

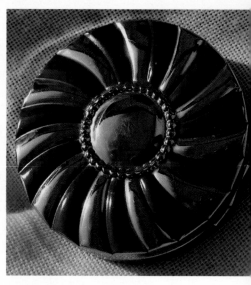

Ritz powder compact. $45-$55.

Red and silver compact, unmarked. $25-$40.

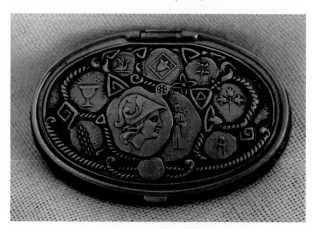

Decorated silver lid on alligator bottom. Could be used for several purposes, including a compact. $50-$75

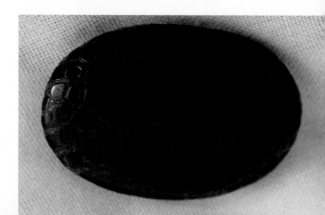

Dyed black alligator bottom.

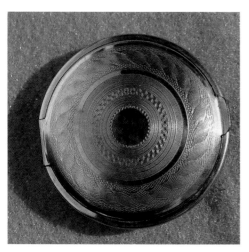

Small, round, silver-colored compact. $20-$25.

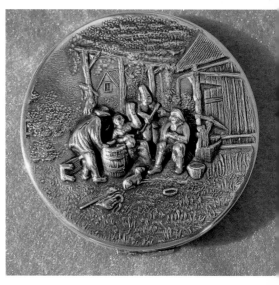

Silver compact made in Denmark. $65-$85.

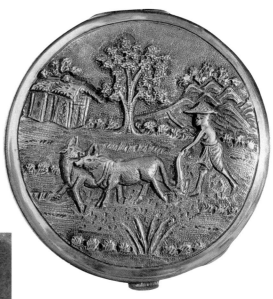

Compact with Oriental scene, unmarked. $60-$75.

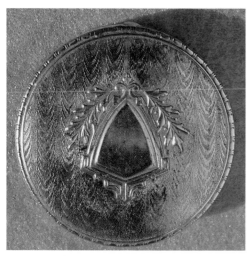

Circa 1920-30 compact. $25-$40.

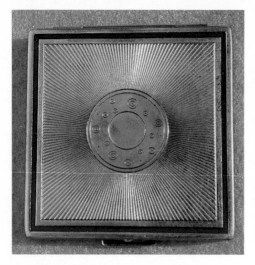

Silver over copper Evening in Paris compact. $20-$30.

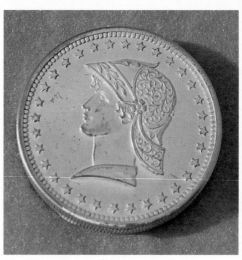

Aluminum compact made to look like coin, unmarked. $100-$125.

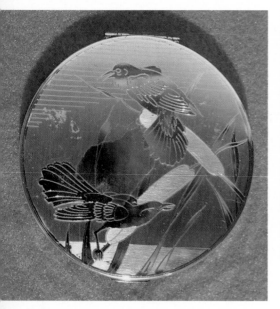

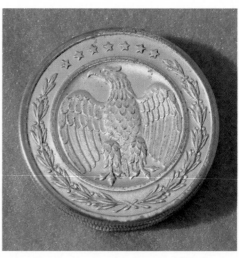

Other side of the compact showing an eagle.

Silver Elgin American compact decorated with birds. $65-$85.

Small, unmarked compact with powder compartment and two mirrors. $20-$25.

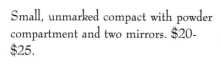

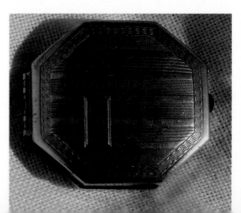

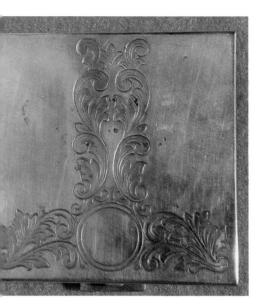

Silver colored top with goldtone decoration and base. $25-$35.

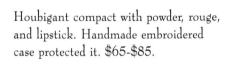

Houbigant compact with powder, rouge, and lipstick. Handmade embroidered case protected it. $65-$85.

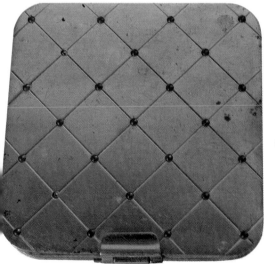

Silver colored metal studded with small green glass. $40-$50.

Small, round compact, girl in Victorian dress. $20-$25.

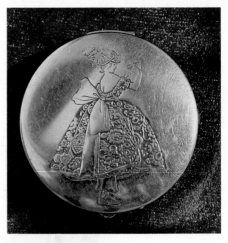

Described on label as French Beauty Box, probably sterling. $95-$125.

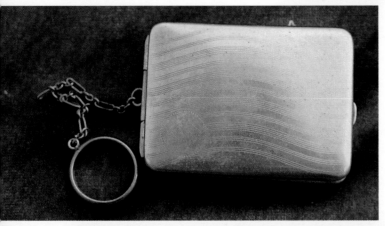

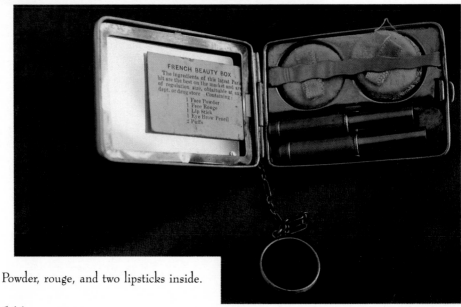

Powder, rouge, and two lipsticks inside.

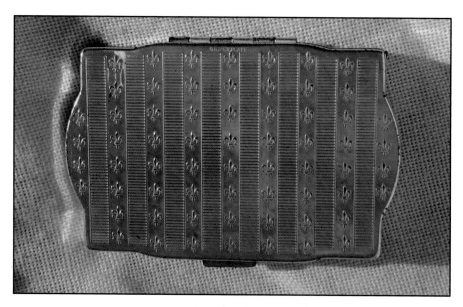

Van Ace silver plated compact. $55-
$75

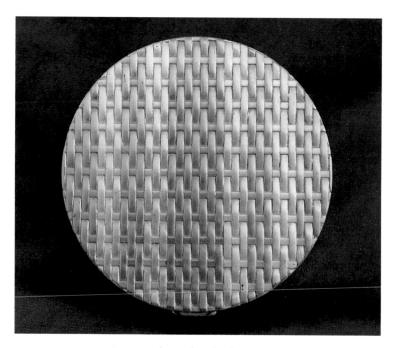

Evans sterling silver basketweave compact. $100-$125.

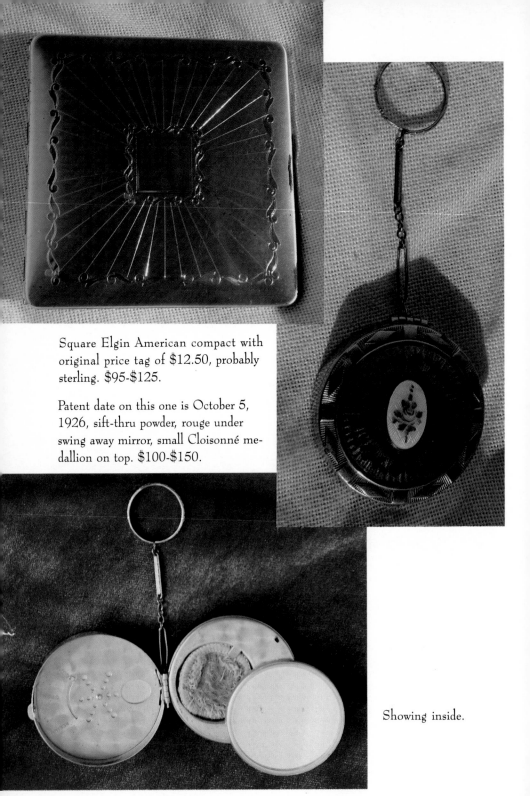

Square Elgin American compact with original price tag of $12.50, probably sterling. $95-$125.

Patent date on this one is October 5, 1926, sift-thru powder, rouge under swing away mirror, small Cloisonné medallion on top. $100-$150.

Showing inside.

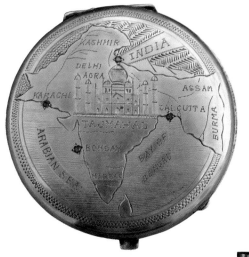

Silver compact with goldtone decorations, from India. $100-$125.

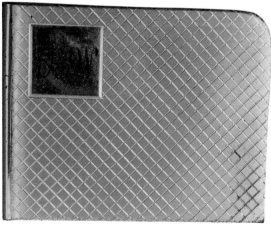

Elgin American sterling compact with goldtone top and place for monogram. $95-$125.

Silver colored compact with goldtone decoration and bottom. $40-$70.

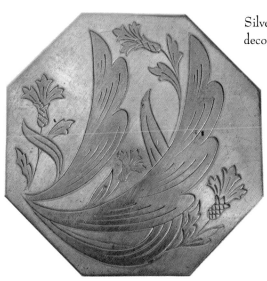

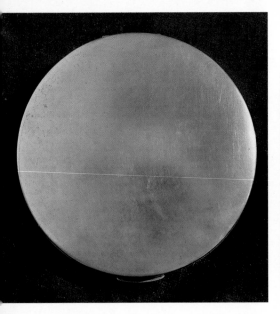

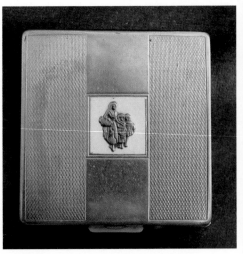

Pilcher silver-plated compact. $75-$95.

Yardley powder compact, white enameled center with figures. $35-$50.

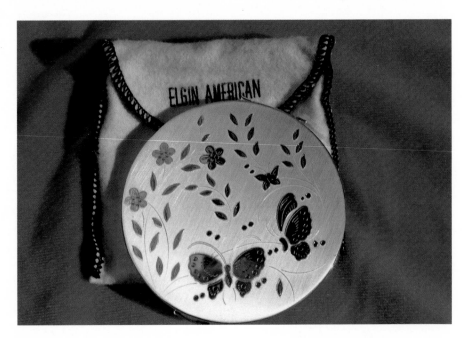

Elgin American silver compact with flowers and butterflies. Still in original box. Also has folder with instructions for applying powder. None in compact but prices are listed. Round, square, and oblong refills with puffs were priced two for $1 while odd shapes were three for $2. $75-$90.

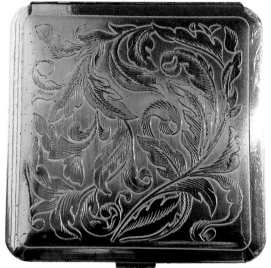

Dorset compact. $50-$65.

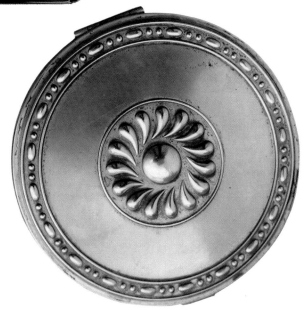

Volupté sterling silver compact. $125-$150.

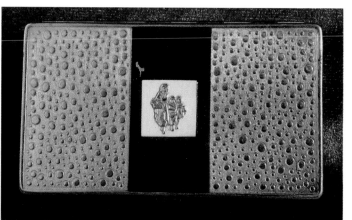

Yardley powder and rouge compact, silver background, black enameled band with goldtone figures. $40-$60.

Chapter Seventeen:
Smoking Accessories

Tobacco was one of the early crops in America. Along with cotton it was one of those crops that made some of the early settlers quite wealthy. Many people, both men and women, tried it with some liking it; others detesting it. One of those women who liked it and continued to smoke her pipe each evening was Rachel Jackson, wife of Andrew Jackson, Seventh president of the United States. She wasn't alone. Many women continued to smoke their pipes well into this century. There were women as well as men who chewed tobacco, and when they made snuff, it was surprising how many women dipped snuff. But it was in the early part of the present century that women really began smoking cigarettes. For the next fifty years at least 75 percent, maybe more, of American women smoked cigarettes. It was considered very fashionable. How could it be otherwise when most of the movie actresses were shown in full page ads not only smoking, but discussing the pleasures of smoking? These same actresses were the ones that young girls admired and wanted to be like; they were the trendsetters so young girls naturally learned to smoke.

And if they were going to smoke, they wanted the feminine touch, a classy container and lighter. During the twenties through the sixties most men used cigarette cases, some rather fancy, but they had a masculine look. The women preferred something more dainty. If they used a separate case, many wanted one with a floral design, mother-of-pearl, or a small case like the snakeskin dyed red or maybe the silver one with hammered design.

Many of the carryalls had a space in the back just for cigarettes. This was an added incentive for women who smoked but didn't want any one to know, and there were many of them. When these women were out on the town and wanted a cigarette, it was so easy to take their carryall and go to the powder room on the pretext of repairing their makeup. They could sneak a smoke while performing that chore. Nobody wanted to take a carryall when they went grocery shopping so the favorite for those trips was the small dainty cases that would fit into a small bag. Larger cases that would fit into larger purses were ideal for traveling.

The cigarette holder seems to have been more important during the Flapper years. Again the women were trying to imitate their favorite actress who so often in the movies used a long cigarette holder. Lighters were also important. Men used masculine lighters that looked very dependable, while women preferred a daintier lighter, usually one that matched her purse, her compact, or her cigarette case. Then there were the musical lighters. Like the musical compacts it is doubtful they were ever used as much as the regular ones, but some woman could have attracted a lot of attention at a party when she used her musical lighter.

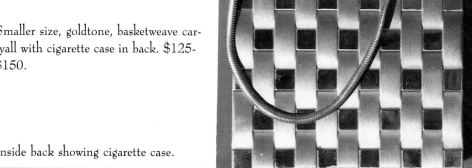

Smaller size, goldtone, basketweave carryall with cigarette case in back. $125-$150.

Inside back showing cigarette case.

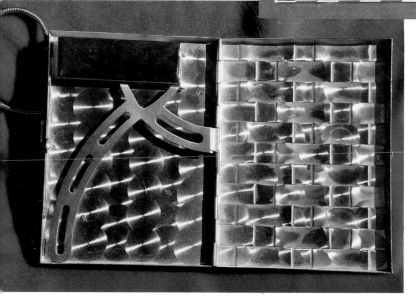

151

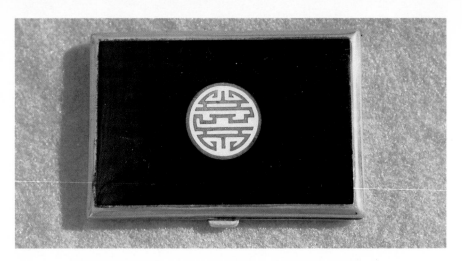

Well-made, lady's size cigarette case, unmarked. $35-$45.

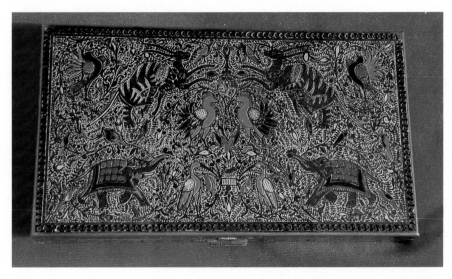

Volupté used this same design on carryalls, compacts, and this cigarette case. $50-$75.

Lady's size Cloisonné cigarette case. $75-$90.

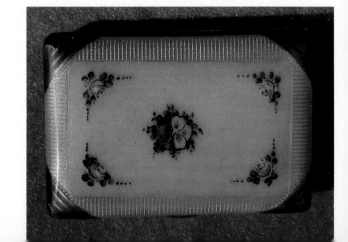

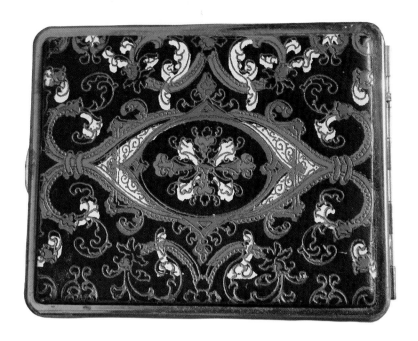

Colorful, leather cigarette case. $45-$65.

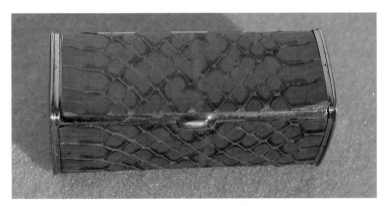

Lady's round, red snakeskin cigarette case. $40-$50.

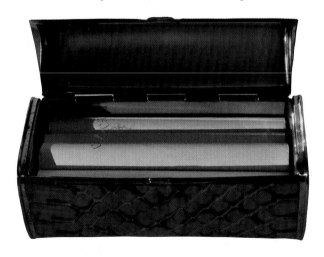

Cigarette case open.

153

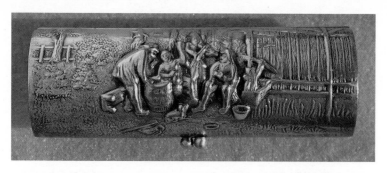

Round, silver cigarette case. Made in Denmark. $75-$90.

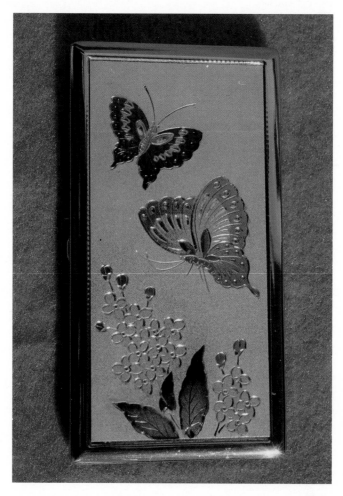

Late cigarette case for king-sized cigarettes decorated with the Art of Chokin, an ancient art form that has been revived. The design is created by etching copper, then gilding it with gold and silver. $65-$85.

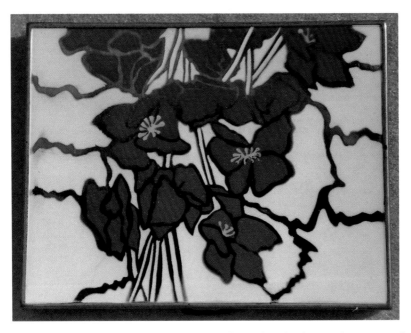

Cigarette case with red flowers outlined in gold on white background. Case marked Alwyn, USA. $50-$65.

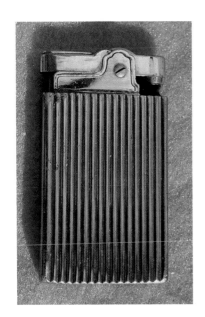

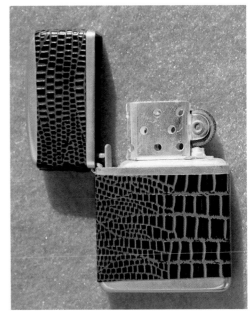

Lady's musical cigarette lighter. $75-$90

Leather-covered cigarette lighter, National Chemsearch on bottom. $25-$35.

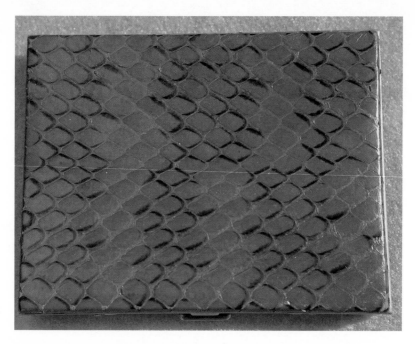

Lady's flat red snakeskin cigarette case.
$45-$65.

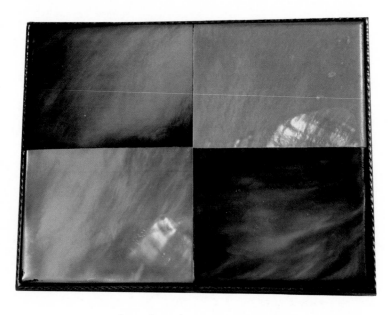

Mother-of-pearl cigarette case, alter-
nating light and dark squares. $75-
$90.

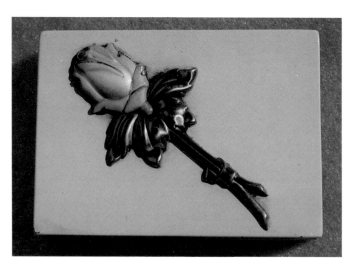

White enameled cigarette case, applied flower with goldtone stem and leaves. $45-$65.

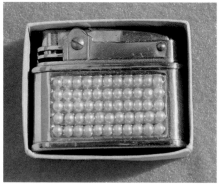

Small, lady's cigarette lighter, 1.25 by 1.75 inches, small imitation pearls on front, Shalco trademark. $25-$35.

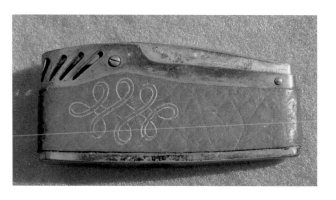

Circa 1950 leather-covered, lady's lighter. Made in Japan. $13-$18.

Information on
Compacts and Their Makers

Compact collectors, like the collectors of all other antiques and collectibles, usually know what they like and want, and search for that particular thing. It may be a style, a color, a maker, or a material. Then there are those who couldn't care less about any thing except what appeals to them. And this could be one of the above, or it could be shape or how the inside is arranged, that is, does it have only powder, or both powder and rouge. Maybe they want powder and lipstick; forget about the rouge. All of these are easy to discover except maybe the maker. Many of the compacts won't have the name of the maker stamped on them. In some cases the name may have been omitted, purposely or otherwise, while in many more the manufacturer's name was only on the puff. But this isn't a done deal today as so many of the original puffs were soiled and replaced with others. Some of the replacements were puffs that could be bought at any so-called dime store. Some of these had names, others didn't, but it was never the original name. Then there were cases where they were replaced by puffs from another compact, made by another maker. Without a name on the compact, or a puff that appears to be the original, it is sometimes next to impossible to say without fear of contradiction that a compact was made by a specific manufacturer. There are exceptions, of course, and one of them is finding the exact compact in an ad or shown in a catalog. Search for compacts made of quality materials and with excellent workmanship, because the names are not always the most important thing. But don't give up on names and trademarks until you have looked carefully as they can be found in the most unusual places, from the sides to the bottom, even under the powder liner. The following is a list of some of the names you are liable to find:

American Beauty
American Maid
Anna Pavlova
Arden, Elizabeth
Armand
Arpels
Artcraft
Avon
Baird North
Barbara Gould
Belle
Blanchette DeCorday
Bree
Campus Makeup
Cara Mia
Cara Noma
Chanel
Chantrey
Charlton
Charles of the Ritz
Cheramy
Colleen Moore
Columbia Fifth Ave.
Coro
Coty
Daniel
Darling
Divine
Djer-Kiss
Dorette
Dorothy Gray
Dorset, 5th Ave.
Dubarry
Dunhill Vanity
Easterling
Elgin American
Embassy
Estee Lauder

Evans
Evening in Paris
Fabergé
Fianceé Woodworth
Flato
Foster
Gainsborough
Gigi
Girey
Givenchy
Gucci
Hammacher Schlemmer
Hampden
Harriet Hubbard Ayers
Hattie Carnegie
Helena Rubenstein
Helene Curtis
Henri Bendel, New York
Henriette
Hollywood
Houbigant
Illinois Watch Case Co.
Jean La Solle
J. M Fisher Co.
Jonteel
K & K
Karess
Kissproof
La Mode
Lady Esther
Lady Lee
Lady Vanity
Langlois
Lederer
Lilly Daché
Lin-Bren
Lovely
Lubin

Lucien Lelong
Lucretia Vanderbilt
Luxor Limited
Majestic
Mara
Marhill
Marlene
Mary Dunhill
Mavco
Mavis
Max Factor
May-Fair
Melba
Mello-Glo
Metalfield
Park & Tilford
Pilcher Manufacturing Co.
Pompeian
Prince Matchabelli
Princess Pat
Quinlan
Revlon
Rex Fifth Avenue
Rex Products Corp.
Richard Hudnut
Ritz

Sam Fink
Schildkraut
Shields
Stadium Girl
Starlet Compact
Stratton
Superb
Tangee
Tre-Jur
Terri Vanities
Tiffany & Co.
Tussy
Unique
Van Cleef & Arpels
Van Ace
Vashé
Volupté Inc.
Wadsworth
Warner of California
Warner of Hollywood
Whiting & Davis Co.
Wiesner of Miami
Woodbury
Yardley
Zell